BACK TO BALANCE:

HEAL YOUR SPINE, HEAL YOUR LIFE

By Raven Sadhaka Seltzer

M.A., E-RYT 500

Second Edition

Published by
Smartbird Publications
P.O. Box 320333
West Roxbury, MA 02132
http://www.selfhealingsolutions.com

Printed in the United States of America, June 2013

ISBN: 978-0-615-81282-3

Library of Congress Catalog Card Number: 2013909269

Cover design by Tricia McMahon
triciamcmahon@comcast.net

First edition published as:
Get Your Low Back on Track: 30 Days to a Healthier Spine

This book is strictly educational, offering information of a general nature to help you in your quest for better spinal health and healthier lifestyle management. It does not provide medical advice or prescribe any technique as a form of treatment for physical or medical problems. Should you use any of the information in this book for yourself, which is your constitutional right, the author and the publisher assume no responsibility for how you understand this material or put it into action. Always seek professional medical assistance for diagnosis and treatment. Use any suggestions in this book as a complement or supplement to physical therapy or therapy that is prescribed.

Acknowledgements

My heartfelt thanks go out to friends and family who have supported me on my life's journey and with this book, through both the original and this latest edition. In particular, thanks to my spiritual teacher, Dr. Barbara DeAngelis, my ALTP & Jyotir Mandala families; my meditation teacher, Dr. Paul Muller-Ortega; my father; my brother Richard for his brainstorming ideas and internet guidance, check out his website at www.samizdat.com; to Karen Kane, a steadfast friend, supporter and yoga student of mine for many years, and many thanks to my wonderful models in this new edition: Stephanie Laverdiere and Marian Murphy.

Thanks so much for Tresca Weinstein for her fine editing skills in the first edition. A special thanks also goes out to Dr. Tom DeMott who read the manuscript of this edition in order to give an endorsement and ended up serving me as an editor, catching some important points that needed clarifying.

I really appreciate Ellen McFarland for her ongoing support of my classes and workshops and for the use of The Center at Westwoods for our photo shoot.

And I have deep gratitude for my yoga teachers and other mentors over many years of study and practice, in particular, Sudha Carolyn Lundeen, Don and Amba Stapleton, Vidya Carolyn Dell'uomo, Devarshi Steven Hartman, Stephen Cope, and Lee Albert. And special thanks to Hasita Agathe Nadai and Brahmani Liebman who started me on my Kripalu yoga journey as I was healing from knee surgery, a low back injury and ultimately avoiding spinal fusion surgery.

Finally, to all of the wonderful students and fellow teachers who have come through my life in these past years, especially within the yoga community that has evolved here in Boston – I've learned so much from each of you.

I dedicate this book to my greatest teachers in this lifetime: my mother, Helen Estes Seltzer, who instilled in me her love of writing, and my father, Dick Seltzer, who has always believed in me and been a great source of inspiration.

TABLE OF CONTENTS

INTRODUCTION TO THE 2ND EDITION

A lot has happened since I wrote and published the first version of this book: the average American is becoming much more savvy about their health and healing and asking more questions. "Holistic healing" and preventative care is becoming more popular and accessible as insurance companies and individuals try to cope with the rising costs of primary medical care and treatment. There is also more public awareness around spinal fusions and their possible risks and long-term effects – word of mouth and first-hand experience has been a powerful source of knowledge.

I have worked with many more private clients and have learned much from their experiences as well as from my own, ongoing maintenance program, as well as a great deal of transformational spiritual work that I have done during this time. I've also worked more with clients dealing with cervical nerve impingement and neuropathy. I'm happy to report that all of the techniques and practices I've laid out in this book work equally well for the cervical/thoracic part of the spine as well as the lumbar spine.

It felt like the right time to review and incorporate the useful feedback I received, and to update and revise the wisdom of this book and program. I was happy to receive the expertise and guidance of other practitioners and mentors whom I greatly admire in putting this new version together.

The original title <u>Get Your Low Back on Track: 30 Days to a Healthier Spine</u> was a good one to start with and get the book out there, but many felt that the title did not speak to the whole program which I offer within these pages. It is not just about healing your physical spine – it is about healing your life simultaneously from the inside out. It is still designed as a 30-day program and I recommend you follow it that way for the most successful results.

Introduction to the First Edition

Welcome to the program and congratulations on taking a positive step forward on your path of healing. You now have in your possession all of the wisdom and knowledge I used to heal my own spine and avoid surgery, as well as my years of experience in sharing these methods, movements, poses and routines with private clients and group classes. It has been very powerful to witness others take initiative on multiple levels and heal themselves completely. I hope to spread this work and wisdom through my book. With the book, you get to have this wisdom at your disposal and to use without leaving your own home.

This program works the way I do: from the premise that knowledge is power and, more specifically, awareness is power. The fact that you are looking for alternative solutions such as this program indicates that you are already aware that in order to heal your lower back, *something must change*, and *you* are the only person who can make that change.

I like to keep things simple and take a holistic approach, so while our goal may be to heal the spine, the entire physical body will be taken into consideration as well as the emotional, psychological, and even spiritual aspects of your life. While you're using this program, I encourage you to learn as much as you can about what's going on with your lower back; ask questions, speak with your medical practitioner, study your x-rays and MRI's; do further research online and find others who are going through a similar situation. Stay open and receive.

Why 30 Days?

It's widely accepted and road-tested that if you can consistently stick to a daily routine for at least 30 days, it is more likely to become a habit. I personally have started many positive habits this way, and that's why I designed this as a 30-day program.

By following the program, you are laying the foundation for your new, healthy spine and your new life. I'll offer facts and statistics as well as anatomy and lifestyle lessons. Each day you will be invited to practice a specific affirmation along with a therapeutic yoga-based movement. You'll find lists of all 30 affirmations and all 30 therapeutic movements in the Appendix; you may want to print these out and carry them around with you, to work or to class. Let the movements turn into a daily routine for you, adding a new one each day. Feel free to mix and match your movements and breath work—some days you may only have time for a 10-minute practice, other days you will have 20 minutes. Any amount of time is better than skipping a day!

I recommend taking the full 30 days to try the whole program rather than speeding through it (though you can certainly read ahead). I've kept the chapters and "assignments" short on purpose—this program is meant to **relieve, energize, and empower you**, not overwhelm you. It's fine to repeat parts of it or do it at a slower pace if you need to as long as you see it through from start to finish at least once.

After 30 days, it's up to you to keep the new routine going, using the book as a reference and resource to come back to. Remember, this is not a "quick fix"—there's no such thing in reality. Work the program and it will work for you.

Building Blocks for Optimal Spinal Health

If you think of your spine as the foundation to your "house" – the body that you have been given to carry around your soul/spirit – remember that when your foundation has problems and weaknesses, it can't support you. This begins to impact many areas of your life. Think of the 30 days and 30 chapters as building blocks of the foundation for this new, healthy house you are creating from the inside out.

To heal yourself on all levels, you need to look carefully at the foundation to find the cracks and degeneration, and then make some new and different choices – to heal the cracks, shore up your support beams, and possibly even remove/replace some emotional and/or psychological blocks.

This book and program is especially designed to help you get to the root of your pain and heal it from the ground up so that your recovery is permanent and that you don't need surgery, or if you've already had the surgery you won't need another.

Here is the basic recipe we will follow:

1) **Get out of pain first.**
2) **Use gentle poses/movements to build flexibility & strength.**
3) **Coordinate breath with movement.**
4) **Use breathing techniques in poses & as a meditation.**
5) **Examine lifestyle, daily habits & nourishment; make adjustments as necessary.**
6) **Use the tools offered in the book to keep track of your progress.**

As you go through the program, feel free to use the journal pages provided in the Appendix or buy your own blank notebook to keep a daily log of thoughts, feelings, habits, changes, diet, and anything else that comes up. Each day, either in the morning or before you go to bed, make some notes about how you're doing. There is no "right" or "wrong" way to do this—it's for your own reference. You can make it as creative or as matter-of-fact as you like. A bullet-point list is fine.

I suggest that you begin your journal with the story of your lower back pain. What exactly happened? What led up to it? Can you pinpoint it? Perhaps a one-time injury or accident? Or did it happen gradually over time? Think of yourself as a detective. Use this exercise not to dwell upon the past, but rather to see if you can learn more about some of your habits and activities, thereby opening the possibility of preventing similar situations from arising in the future. And remembering the ingredients you use that lead to your full recovery. There will also be various charts and questionnaires to fill out as you go through the book – please do them in order and don't jump ahead. There is a reason for their order here. At the very end of the book, I have provided a blank monthly chart to copy, based on the practices you will establish – to help you keep the process going..

If you are on prescription pain medication and/or anti-inflammatory medication, please consult with your physician before stopping them or beginning this program. Some of the restorative poses could bring significant pain relief – I know they did for me – but this program is not meant to be a substitute for medical evaluation or treatment.

I will offer you Complimentary Alternative Modalities (CAMs) and alternate ways of looking at and dealing with your pain and recovery process. And please remember, it will most likely take a combination of therapies, unique to each person, to make a full recovery, so stay open to other complimentary alternatives. Here are a few worth incorporating and investigating: chiropractic, network spinal analysis, acupuncture, massage therapy, reiki, positional therapy, craniosacral therapy and reflexology. There are a number of practitioners in the Northeastern U.S. listed in my resources section. Make sure you look up credentials and get personal recommendations from others if you live in another state or country.

Lifestyle management

Throughout this program, you will find easy yoga and/or therapeutic movement exercises to heal the low back, usually one for each day and chapter. These moves and poses are designed to gently stretch and strengthen the muscles. You will also be offered the opportunity to evaluate your lifestyle, eating habits and body mechanics as well as some ideas for changing current practices that may be thwarting your healing process. Ultimately, re-conditioning the mind and healing yourself energetically is an absolute necessity if you want to keep prevent re-injuring the same area or another part of your physical body.

Deep breathing and slowing down in general are also encouraged. Get into the habit of stopping to take a breath before you move or act, before you open your mouth to say something – this can benefit your life in so many ways and allows a moment to ground and get a different perspective on a situation. We'll talk more about breath in the first few chapters.

Please note: If you have an acute situation with your back, it is always best to consult your primary care physician first, have X-rays taken, MRI's if necessary, and to receive a diagnosis from them before moving ahead with this program. If you have a chronic condition and have already been through that process, use your own best judgment about implementing this program. If you have any questions or doubts about proceeding, please consult your medical provider.

A contract with yourself

On the next page is a contract I would like you to read, sign and date before you begin the program. Keep it on hand—or for additional reinforcement, you may want to mail it to yourself and be surprised when you find it in your mailbox in a few days.

Remember, you deserve to be healthy and well. This is your natural state. You are capable of alleviating your pain and healing your low back or neck issues. I send you many blessings on your healing path as we begin this work together!

Take the first step in faith.
You don't have to see the whole staircase,
just take the first step.
—Dr. Martin Luther King, Jr.

<u>Holistic Healing Contract</u>

I, _____, am committed to completing this 30-day program and all of the exercises included in order to develop strength and flexibility and create long-lasting spinal health.

I, _____, am committed to identifying and releasing any lifestyle habits that do not serve me in the process of healing my neck and/or back issues.

I, _____, am committed to identifying what nourishes me, my healing process, my relationships, and my True Self (as opposed to my ego-mind).

I, _____, am committed to the practice of releasing fear and negativity from my life and from my body.

I, _____, am committed to the practice of honoring and loving myself as I explore the self-care practices introduced in the program.

I, _____, am committed to directing my conscious focus toward healing my spinal issues. I recognize that affirmations can help me do this.

I, _____, am committed to re-directing my subconscious mind with the use of guided visualizations and meditations provided with the program.

_____
(Signature)

_____
(Date)

Honor yourself for taking a bold and powerful step toward healing your spine and accepting responsibility and accountability for your own progress. If you forget why you're doing this, re-read your contract to remember.

(Make a copy of this, fill it out and sign it. Keep it posted in clear view for the next 30 days.)

Materials needed for your 30 days:

- Yoga sticky mat, exercise mat or yoga rug (not essential, but it could be used to define your "healing space" at home (i.e., setting boundaries with partners, roommates, kids)
- A yoga strap or long belt, or two men's ties tied together – get creative!
- A foam block or thick, sturdy cushion (not too big) that gives some resistance
- A blanket, cushion or yoga bolster for support under the knees (or a nice bulky pillow)
- A small towel or fleece blanket for padding under the head
- A straight-backed chair for certain poses
- Journaling pages are provided in the back or you can buy yourself a blank notebook or journal to write in each day.
- An open mind

(I recorded a CD of Guided Visualizations for Deep Healing which can be used throughout your healing journey. It can be purchased separately through my website: www.selfhealingsolutions.com.. The CD offers added relaxation benefits, however, it is not a requirement for successfully completing the program.)

CHAPTER 1:   MOBILITY AND STABILITY

DAY 1

Motion is the lotion, and motion creates healing.

In western medical terms when talking about the spine, these two terms "*mobility*" and "*stability*" can seem to be at odds and this immediately set up an "all or nothing" view of how to proceed with treatment. It is implied that a patient needs to choose one over the other and stability is usually what is recommended more strongly—hence the spike in spinal surgeries in the past ten to fifteen years. I am happy to say that this has been evening out and more orthopedists and even orthopedic surgeons are opening to alternative and holistic approaches, with surgery being a last resort.

The first thing that you need to know is that it is possible to have both mobility and stability in the spine, as long as your condition is not too far along. There may have to be a compromise in that case, but there are still options. Many times, the bodily systems and functions , in this case, the muscular system, are overlooked or forgotten, when in reality they are our first line of healing tools and defense against further damage to discs and vertebrae.

There are places in the body and the spine in particular that require a certain degree of mobility in order for the joint or the extremity to be used effectively, and this mobility contributes to the stability of these areas as well. These qualities are both very important and you need to know what you are getting into before you begin making sacrifices and choose to go under the knife.

If you lock two vertebrae up with each other permanently, no matter what materials are used, this immediately creates a ripple effect throughout the rest of the spine. All of the sudden your other vertebrae, especially the two directly bookending this area, will now take on more work to make up for the fusion and permanent rigidity created.

If you think about any moving, living organism, system or even a machine, the same would be true -- you stop two moving parts from moving together and prevent them from ever doing so again. It's like 2 employees from your company get laid off and the whole department is affected and everyone feels the sting – more work, less hands.

The Most Common Conditions

If there is weakness and pain in the spine (usually cervical or lumbar) along with any disc injury, stenosis, slippage of the vertebrae and/or **degenerative disc disease** (the wearing down of disc height between the vertebrae), an orthopedic surgeon will most likely recommend "stabilizing" or fusing" vertebrae together. Sometimes, if the degeneration of the bone is extensive, surgery may be your only option, but any strengthening of the spinal muscles and stretching out of the hip muscles will still benefit you greatly, pre- and post-surgery.

If you have neck pain or discomfort, the same principles apply – gentle movement and stretching will help to release the impingement of the nerve, the pain will dissipate and then you can begin your healing process, realigning your posture and your neck.

The most common problem is the classic "pinched nerve in C7." Cervical 7 is the last vertebrae of the neck and T1 is the first thoracic vertebra; between them the 8th cervical nerve threads through and often gets compressed. The causes can be anything from sleeping on a pillow that is too soft, to spending too many hours hunched up at the computer screen, to lifting a heavy baby or object repeatedly or incorrectly. The effects are usually pain along the back of the upper arm and/or numbness in the hands or fingers.

If you reach around right now and feel down, just below the curve of your neck, there will be a bony bump sticking out. If you reach your head forward, it will become more pronounced. This is normal – it's the spinous process of your 7th cervical vertebra sticking out.

What is a "fusion?"

Fusion is an invasive surgical procedure in which two or more vertebrae are joined together, that is, permanently "fused" to immobilize an area of the spine. Bone grafts, titanium plates or bars and screws, are secured on and around the affected area during surgery. This surgery is often recommended for people with cervical disc herniation, degenerative disc disease, and/or spondylolisthesis (one vertebra slips forward over the one beneath it).

The spine is designed to be mobile; fusing vertebrae together locks part of the spine in permanent immobility. This locking in one area inhibits movement in other areas of the spine as well. In addition, it creates extreme wear and tear on the bone and discs above and below the area of the fusion, because they are trying to over-compensate for the area that is now locked in place.

For an excellent X-ray example of a spinal fusion, please see: http://www.laserspineinstitute.com/spinal_orthopedic_procedures/spinal__fusion (I don't necessarily recommend this company's services or methods or its doctors, but the website is informative.) Also, here is a very sobering look at "Hardware for Back Surgery," where you can see samples of the bars, screws and "cages" that are used in a fusion: http://machinedesign.com/article/hardware-for-back-surgery-0112

Since the pain and symptoms of degenerative disc disease all stem from nerve impingement, I believe that most of the time, **gentle movement and deep breathing can relieve pain and create healing** or play a large part in these processes.

What to consider before surgery

Any permanent immobilization of the vertebral column is a very serious matter and should be considered carefully. As technology improves, spinal fusions are becoming easier to perform. The good news is that arthroscopic techniques are making this surgery less invasive, but the downside of the improved technology is that these procedures are being recommended more readily as a "quick fix". Sometimes there is no alternative to surgery, but a number of clients have come to me with more problems than they had before having the surgery.

If a doctor does recommend spinal surgery to you, do yourself a favor and get two or three opinions before you make a decision—and try other alternatives first before going under the knife. Even if you end up having surgery, this program will still be a great resource for stretching and strengthening and may shorten your recovery time; you'll recover your muscle tone and full range of motion more quickly.

Fusing vertebrae together cannot be reversed and eventually bone will grown over the metal bars or bone graft used, leading to bone spurs, arthritis and stenosis. According to statistics, about one quarter of all grafts do not take and it is necessary for another fusion to be performed. Less than half of conventional surgeries, including fusions, succeed in alleviating the pain and symptoms and the healing phase may be long and painful.

If you are not incredibly overweight and without other health issues, there are now some minimally invasive alternative techniques which are developing and may be less risky than the traditional fusion surgery.

In 2001 I was diagnosed with grade 2 spondylolisthesis in my L5 verte-brae and fusion was strongly recommended. I was told that I would not be able to walk upright without pain unless I went through with this surgery. I am so glad I did not take this path and instead sought out the wisdom of yoga and Ayurveda. This is me today, working on my wheel pose:

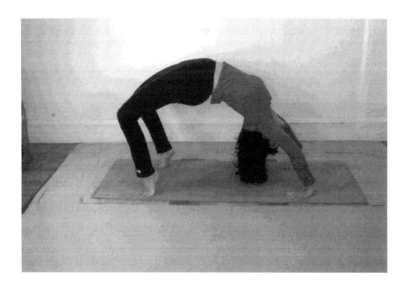

Eventually, I will be able to get my heels down to the floor and shift more of my upper body weight over my shoulders, elbows and hands. This is an amazing turnaround for me from where I was at the time of my diagnosis. I can't guarantee that my book will get you to this place – I had many years of yoga practice and training before coming into wheel pose – but you will definitely ex-perience more flexibility and relief if you follow this program.

My pain is gone, but it did not happen overnight with any magical potions, or wishful thinking and it does require my constant vigilance: daily stretching and strengthening with yoga, movement and pranayama (breath/energy work) as well as maintaining a healthy diet and lifestyle. I made a personal choice not to follow a doctor's recommendation and I am glad of it, but this is serious business and you need to consider all of your options before making any decisions.

As I mentioned before, sometimes there is no alternative to fusion, for example, if you have a spinal bone deformity from birth or in extreme cases where the bone loss is so significant that you must have help to stabilize the spine. However, I personally know a number of people who had the cervical fusion procedure and are quite unhappy; they still have pain and now their range of motion is virtually nonexistent, so they have less ability to relieve their own discomfort and they have become more reliant on pain medications. I'm told that the cervical fusion is like being in a very strong neck brace…for the rest of your life. Please do lots of research and weigh all of your options before going through with any surgery. Everyone's situation is unique.

My offering for you here is to use movements, breathing, lifestyle management, and ergonomic tips to avoid surgery if at all possible. I believe that yoga and other forms of strengthening and stretching have shown that mobility is very important, if not essential for the health of the joints in the body. It keeps our bodies supple and in combination, can easily be used to alleviate pain.

AFFIRMATION: I AM FULLY PRESENT AND GROUNDED IN THIS MOMENT.

POSE: MODIFIED VIPARITA KARANI (LEGS UP OVER A CHAIR, OR UP AGAINST THE WALL)

- Place a straight-backed chair onto your mat or a rug (or put your mat in front of a sofa or armchair)
- Lie down with your legs extended toward the chair.
- Now swing both legs up over the seat of the chair and bring your lower legs to rest on the chair seat.
- You may want to use a small towel or cushion under the back of the head for comfort.**
- Your feet may stick through the space between the back and seat of the chair. Inch your hips up toward the legs of the chair until you feel your low back is comfortable.
- Stay here for 3 to 5 minutes, or longer if you can.
- The chair helps take a great deal of pressure off the lower back.
- You can use this position to relax in each day after your movement workouts.

**Support the head and neck with a soft, folded blanket or thin pillow. If you have cervical issues then this is even more important for you

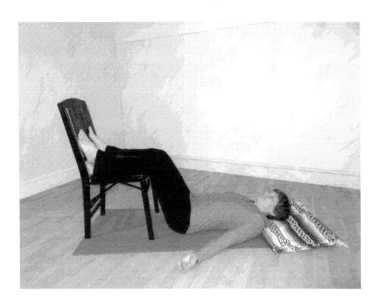

CHAPTER 2: THE SPINE: AN ENGINEERING WONDER

DAY 2

It's a marvel to look at an image of the spine -- this curved bony structure that holds us upright -- and realize that this structure creates the core of our foundation. And that if we pay attention to our daily habits and posture, the spine will stay in good shape and support us faithfully.

The vertebrae play an intricate role in a much larger tapestry. Remember that old song "The backbone's connected to the hipbone"? This chain is actually more like a circle or cycle that we will travel around, taking apart and putting back together your lower back and your life. The spine offers us support, mobility and protection of the spinal cord.

Your spine is a very complex engineering miracle that allows you movement, the ability to carry your body upright against the forces of gravity, and the protection of your spinal cord and nerves.
– Dr. Jeri Anderson

The health of the spine and the entire body depends on getting enough oxygen through the breath, getting the proper nutrients through food, making smart lifestyle choices and changes and learning to move and breathe our bodies in therapeutic ways. Coordinating breath with movement is one way to become more aware the connection between the mental, emotional and physical bodies. Self-care, nourishment, and lifestyle are also interdependent.

We have choices about almost every one of these pieces of the puzzle— how much or how little we do or eat or sleep or move. Perhaps the only wild card is oxygen—we aren't usually able to control how much O_2 is in each of the environments we enter. But that makes it all the more important to maximize your lung power, capacity and the ability of your body to use the oxygen you breathe in.

Committing to this program for 30 days is a perfect opportunity to increase your awareness of the spine and your whole body as a miracle machine of sorts. The more you can bring your focus inside, back to your own center, the more deep healing you will experience.

"Holistic" healing is about healing from the inside out; bringing yourself back to wholeness by connecting the inner and outer worlds. There are so many other factors involved in maintaining good spinal health. The physical aspect is just one level. Your injury and recovery hinge on this concept of connection and creating wholeness—it's not just about healing your lower back.

Some other ideas for this 30-day time you have -- take a "media break." Turn the television off for a while. Read a book, spend time with loved ones. Do your yoga and breathing. Media overload keeps our brains buzzing, making it much more difficult to explore awareness. Look at other things in your environment and how you react to them. It is possible to change and re-learn more useful skills for dealing with the stress in our lives and in the world around us. We will get into lifestyle choices in more depth in a later chapter. In the meantime, keep in mind that it's always best to inquire within first.

AFFIRMATION: I GRATEFULLY TAKE RESPONSIBILITY FOR MY HEALTH AND WELL-BEING.

MOVEMENT: PELVIC TILTING.

- Lie down on your back. Close your eyes.
- Bend your knees to bring the soles of your feet onto the floor.
- Practice stacking the joints. Feel the ankles under the knees.
- On an inhale, roll your tailbone forward and down into the floor, feeling an arch forming in the small of your back.
- As you exhale, slowly flatten the small of your back against the floor, curling the tailbone up.
- Your hips may lift slightly, but it's not necessary to make any effort to do so.
- Keep this movement going, slow and steady, for about 10 breaths. Imagine you are riding a wave of breath; allow your lower back to be fluid.
- Keep eyes closed or use a soft gaze for maximum healing effect.

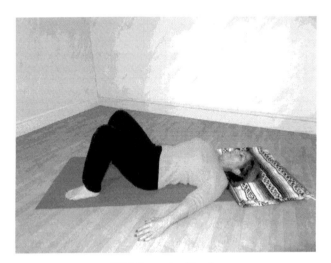

Slightly arched back

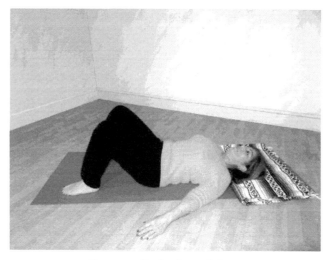

Return to flat back, neck long

POSE: SAVASANA

This is a relaxation pose that you can use each day at the end of your movement workouts.

- Lie flat on your back, adding a bolster, pillow, or rolled-up blanket under the knees, and any other props you need.
- Let the head, torso, legs, & arms all be heavy. Let your body melt into the floor. Rest here for 5 to 10 minutes.

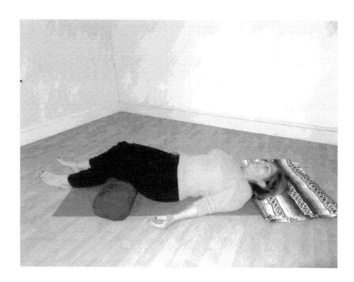

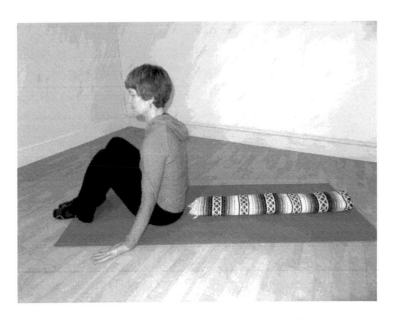

You can also use a blanket roll under the spine & head.

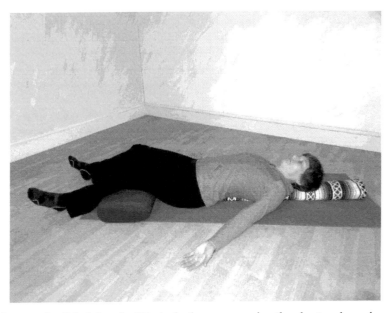

This is great for dislodging the C7 pinched nerve, opening the chest and moving your spine and ribcage back into alignment.

CHAPTER 3: WHO'S DRIVING YOUR CAR?

DAY 3

Think of your body a vehicle that carries around your soul, spirit, chi, life force, or whatever you prefer to call it. Your body, like a car, must be well maintained in order to work properly and carry you through life. It needs proper rest, nourishment, warming up, cooling down, exercise – a lot like letting the engine run and taking it for long, leisurely drives. And just like an auto mobile, any extreme acceleration, slamming on the brakes or hard turns to the wheel puts extra wear and tear on your car, it's motor and different parts.

So, who is driving this car-body of yours? Are you connected to your body or are you in your head most of the time, thinking about the past or the future? If you can become aware of when you are neglecting your own needs and bring yourself back to awareness, this the first step in any healing process. Usually it takes a painful sensation or situation for us to wake up to this awareness.

The Cruise-Control Epidemic

I frequent a healthy restaurant not far from my home that lets you design your own stir-fry; you select the fresh vegetables you want, put them in a bowl, and hand it to the chef. You tell the chef what else you'd like in your stir-fry—brown rice, chicken, teriyaki sauce—and he follows the order as you dictate it. The last two times I went there, a different young man has waited on me. The first time I asked for chicken, but when got my dish back to the table, there was no chicken in the dish. I took it back. He apologized; I could tell he was preoccupied and his body was here and speaking to me, but energetically, he was miles away.

The next time, I asked for teriyaki sauce on the side. This time I paid attention and noticed that the kid was flipping the stir-fry pan, but his mind was miles away. He added teriyaki sauce to the bowl automatically even though I had requested it on the side. These are just small and innocent examples from everyday life that we can all relate to and have also done ourselves. Whenever we make this choice though, we are essentially allowing someone else to drive our car, our body.

When you switch over to "cruise control," or automatic pilot, you disengage the body-mind connection right away. You project your mind into past or future, but you leave your body in the present to deal with the consequences. In doing this, you run the risk of serious injury to yourself and others because you are not paying attention to what is happening in the present, not listening to messages that your body or the universe may be giving you.

This is not a good strategy for living in the world, or for protecting the lower back. Injuries happen in the most mundane situations because we "just weren't thinking," or maybe we were thinking too much and forgot to take a moment to pause and breathe. Whenever you do this, you are essentially taking your hands off the wheel.

As a culture, we Americans tend to have trouble focusing on the present, and it's no wonder. Life is complicated enough without 400 channels to choose from, laptops, cell phones, GPS, PlayStation and Xbox games, etc. Then there's the pressure to have the right house in the right neighborhood and the right car in the driveway, and to send our children to the right schools and make enough money to keep them there. Life is hard before you even get to your relationships with partners, family, coworkers, and friends—if you even have time for interacting. We are constantly trying to cram in three days' worth of activities and work into 24 hours.

We are generally sleeping less and not very deeply. We rush everywhere, so our nourishment habits are quite poor. If you live in a big city, your situation is likely even more intensified, and when we do try to "get healthy," the most popular and accessible choices are the extremes—power yoga, spinning, extreme sports. When we jump into situations which our bodies are not ready to handle, without the correct guidance and warm-ups, exercise can actually harm us.

And most of the time our injuries have nothing to do with sports or working out. It just takes a moment: that questionable move -- contorting your body to reach something or bending over to lift something that's too heavy with no support and locked knees. All of the sudden your back is gonzo! Ouch, what happened?

Try this little exercise when you have a few moments to yourself to help you stay more conscious and in the moment:

Find a quiet space. Sit comfortably on the edge of a chair, close your eyes, and breathe in and out through your nose. Feel your feet flat on the floor. Notice how your whole torso expands and contracts as you breathe in and out. If your mind wanders, count how long it takes for the breath to come in and fill your body and then count your exhale too. Focus on your breath like this for three minutes.

Open your eyes. Notice how you feel. Keep that sense of presence in each moment – you can use the breath at any time, eyes open or closed, to connect to your own center.

When you pay this kind of attention to your body and reconnect with sensation and emotion, it's highly unlikely that you will injure yourself or your low back.

Control

We like to focus on other people's lives and even attempt to control them, especially when our own lives are spinning out of control. Look at the number of reality TV shows on these days. It used to be soap operas. A great many people in this country give more time to their favorite reality programs or soaps than they do to their own self-care or their family's well-being. Let's begin to counteract that external focus.

YOUR TASK FOR THE DAY

Focus on the present moment: When you find yourself projecting into the future (worrying about where you have to go) or the past (worrying about what just happened or obsessing about something that happened years ago), take a deep breath and on the exhale, let go. Release the thought and come back into your body using the breath. Notice your rhythm as you breathe in and out. Notice any sensations present in the body..Close the eyes if possible

This is an easy way to begin a meditation practice.

AFFIRMATION: I AM ENOUGH—I HAVE ALL I NEED.

POSE: HALF FROG

- Lie down on your stomach, rest your forehead on the backs of your hands or turn one cheek to the side. Tune into what position feels best for your neck.
- Slide one knee up towards your shoulder; stop where you need to and keep the bend in the knee.
- For large bellies or breasts, get creative and comfortable! Position pillows, blankets or cushions under your head or torso.
- Stay here for at least a few minutes, breathing in and out and feeling the release in the lower back and hip area.
- This pose is great for releasing the gluteus medius (connecting pelvis to femur bone) and piriformis (connects the sacrum to the femur bone) muscles in particular.

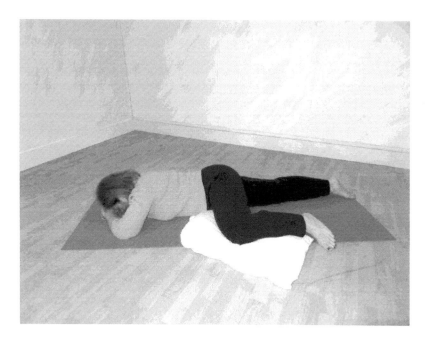

Half Frog with pillow under knee

CHAPTER 4: CONNECTING TO THE BREATH

DAY 4

You can live for weeks without food and for days without water, but without oxygen you would be dead in minutes.

The breath is your connection between the external and internal worlds. Breath is taken in as oxygen and exhaled as carbon dioxide and nitrogen, both waste products. In the simple act of breathing, your body becomes a laboratory. A biochemical reaction is created by respiration. With each breath you inhale and exhale, you heal. It's as simple as that. And there are no adverse side effects to breathing more deeply, just beneficial ones! The exhale is just as important as the inhale – we must get those toxins out of the lungs.

There are three ways in which the breath directly promotes healing:

1) The motion of breathing in and out creates an expansion/contraction in the body that in turn creates a massaging action, relaxing the internal organs and releasing toxins from the kidneys and adrenals and tension from the muscles, tendons, and ligaments. Deep breathing also massages your heart, improves

circulation and aids digestion. It can also help the lower back as the gentle movement of inhale and exhale moves the vertebrae and massages the surrounding muscles, tendons, ligaments, and tissue.

2) The simple act of deepening the breath promotes healing. Deliberate breathing changes your physiology. The deeper the breath, the more oxygen comes into your body and consequently, more oxygen ends up in the blood stream and the cells. Healthy cells require a steady flow of oxygen.

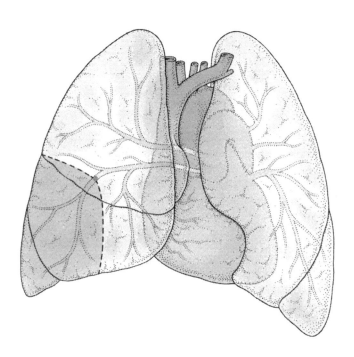

Front view of heart and lungs

The breath is an essential part of health and healing that is generally ignored and/or just not considered important by the medical community (except after you have had surgery and you have to work at getting your oxygen levels back up again).

If you look at the anatomical drawing on the previous page, you'll notice the heart is located in between the lobes of the lungs. With each deep breath we have the ability to literally give the heart a massage. Most physical therapists don't realize that yoga is at the root of their work. Many of the exercises and movements are identical to yoga except that yoga emphasizes the breath and teaches you how to breathe *with* movement. Breath and movement are a powerful combination when used mindfully, deliberately, with focus and compassion. The results will enhance your overall well-being, in addition to healing your physical body.

Many of your internal organs are also massaged by deep, slow, long breaths in and out -- the diaphragm pushes down on the inhale, compressing the intestines and abdominal organs, while creating more space for heart and lungs . On the exhale the diaphragm releases, the lungs empty out and everything moves back into its place. We'll talk more about the diaphragm and the muscles of respiration in Chapter 10.

As I am fond of telling my students and clients, any time you sit quietly or lie down and breathe in and out slowly and deeply, you are doing yoga! If you think about it, we could easily "do yoga" in this way, all day long, every day.

3) Deep breathing also calms the central nervous system (the brain, spinal cord, and nerves), thereby making it a natural pain reliever. Space is created—the spine elongates on an inhale. Space allows for release and relaxation, alleviating compression. The exhale is a release and a letting go.

The inhalation and exhalation process is a three-dimensional action. You can feel this movement prominently in different variations of Child Pose. Notice the breath expanding the front, sides, and back of your body. Think of your torso as a balloon inflating and then deflating.

If we inhale with intention, we are able to increase that expansion. You will notice a lift of the ribcage and an opening of the chest as the spine elongates. By this action, we create space—or more accurately, "reclaim" space in the body. This space is always there, ready to be accessed; it's up to us to sit up, un-hunch our shoulders, open the chest, and allow more breath to flow in.

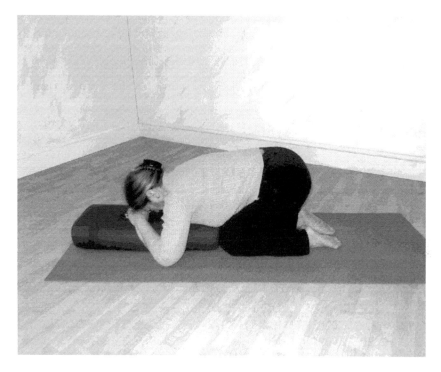

Supported Child Pose using a bolster

Deep breathing has an incredible effect on all systems of the body. Remember: the exhalation is just important as the inhalation. It is essential for the lungs to expel all of the toxins—that is what the exhale helps us to do.

Physically, on an exhale, we feel the chest, torso, and back body deflate. As the belly draws in, see if you can notice and then emphasize pulling the belly button back towards the spine. This is very helpful in clearing out the last of the breath. The inhale will naturally come in again. The exhale empties the belly and lungs and makes it easier to feel the muscles engage, particularly those in the abdominal area.

Nasal Breathing versus Mouth Breathing

The primary passage for the inhale should always be the nostrils. The nose, the nostrils and nose hairs were specifically designed to take in the breath, filter it and send it down into the lungs in the most concentrated way. Simply put, mouth breathing is a poor substitute and nowhere near as effective – it is a good secondary passage, if the nasal passages are congested, but regular mouth breathing is not recommended as it doesn't not bring enough oxygen into the lungs to expand them fully. The rest of the bodily systems are affected from there. The breath and oxygen contain our life force energy (prana) and we want do everything we can to cultivate that.

From my own personal experience as well as working with an elderly and senior population for quite some time, I have observed that mouth-breathers are frequently fatigued and have a hard time getting going in the morning. When I work with them to focus on nasal breathing, especially if they have conditions like Congestive Heart Failure and Diabetes, I have witnessed the positive impact it has on their lives – better energy and circulation, sharper senses and mental clarity, less fluid pooling in the lungs and ankles and overall a stronger immune system.

I do not know if medical studies have been done around this, but it makes sense since the heart is between the lungs and the two systems/organs are so intimately connected to and dependent upon each other. The heart is a muscle and a pump for the blood, but the lungs do not have any muscle – they must be filled up with enough air to properly oxygenate the blood. Cells need good levels of oxygen to stay healthy.

The exhale is a different story – a nasal exhale is fine and usually the most desirable for meditation and yogic movement, but there are definitely times when deliberate exhaling through the mouth is a great thing to do – especially when releasing with a movement and making a therapeutic "ha" sound as you let go of tension in the body. The exhale through the mouth can offer a more complete emptying out of the lungs and that's a good thing – you want to get as much carbon dioxide out of the system as possible: this is harmful the waste product that is left over from the metabolic reactions in the body.

If you are more inclined towards mouth-breathing, it may be the result of discomfort with nasal breathing if you are frequently congested (a great reason to try using a neti pot or nasal rinse cup), or this may be rooted in primal needs and fears: the need to survive and/or the fear of being overwhelmed and "drowning" in emotions.

In the Chinese Medicine system, the lungs are believed to be where we hold our grief. When we try to control our emotions, we usually cut our breath short; we don't want to fill up those lungs, we don't want to feel too much because we are terrified of the idea of feeling too much and losing control. Of course, when you do take a deep nasal breath, it provides an excellent way to feel, move through and let go of emotion. Holding your breath and holding yourself back from breathing fully can actually bring on illness and disease.

Where cells get enough oxygen, cancer will not, cannot occur."

--Dr. Otto Warburg, Nobel Prize Winner

AFFIRMATION: I BREATHE IN AND EXPAND, I BREATHE OUT AND RELEASE MORE TENSION. I ALLOW THE BREATH TO MOVE ME AND MY SPINE IN HEALTHY WAYS.

POSE: SUPPORTED CHILD POSE (SEE PHOTO ON PAGE 4)

* Find a comfortable way to sit back on your heels.

- You may need props—a bolster or blanket to stretch out across, and rest on the heels; and/or a small towel or padding under the tops of the feet.
- Lean forward and let your arms be in front of you, hands together.
- Let your forehead rest either on your stacked fists or on the backs of your hands (you may also rest your forehead on a block or cushion).
- Remind yourself that no holding is necessary, no muscles are needed to hold you here, and find a way to create that ease in your body.
- Breathe into the back body and on each exhale release into your child pose.
- This is a wonderful resting pose for transitions between movements and also stimulates the third eye/pineal gland.

**This is another great pose for cervical nerve impingement – bring hands up under the head (or stack your fists) and rest it there. Let the head be heavy and completely relaxed – this will help to release more tension in the neck and shoulder blades and upper back.

CHAPTER 5: BREATHE AND MOVE

DAY 5

Now that we've discussed the importance of the breath, let's look at the essential connection between breath and movement. We naturally breathe in and out all of the time—it is involuntary; we don't have to think about it, it just happens. But we can choose to breathe deliberately and to use the breath to bring more mindfulness to our movement—not just in the healing process, but in everyday life.

INHALE = EXPAND, LIFT, EXERT ENERGY
EXHALE = RELEASE, SINK, LET GO OF TENSION

We can use the breath to help us move up and down and side to side; to lift the weight of a limb or larger area of the body, and release it back down. It turns out that coordinating breath with movement is a very natural thing to do.

Even if you are in great pain, gentle, slow, deep breaths will most certainly be a relief. If all you can do for 30 days is lie on your back and do three-part breaths and some gentle pelvic tilting, you will still notice a difference. Your spine will gently realign itself.

To experience this right now, lie down on your back. Use any props you need to be comfortable. Take a deep breath into your belly and feel the breath expand into the back of the lungs and all the way down into the lower spine. The spine extends and flattens a bit when you take a nice, full, deep breath. If you place your hands gently on your belly, you will feel it rise up as your diaphragm pushes down and then lower down again as you exhale out.

AFFIRMATION: I RIDE THE WAVE OF MY BREATH AND LET IT GUIDE MY MOVEMENTS.

BREATH: THREE-PART BREATH

- In seated pose or lying down with support, practice slowly taking breath in through the nose and let the belly fill up like a balloon.
- Let the air expand up and out into the rib cage. Feel the sides and back and front of your torso open and expand.
- Let the breath come into the upper chest just a bit.
- Exhale the opposite way out—first the upper chest contracts, then the rib cage draws back in, and finally the belly button draws back to the spine as the last bit of air is released through the nose.
- Think about a breath infusing your entire body, filling you up from the soles of your feet all the way up to the crown of your head, like a wave washing through you.
- Then imagine the exhale as the breath leaving your entire body, clearing the path for a new inhalation to follow.
- Remember, the exhalation is just as important as the inhalation!

MOVEMENT: CAT/DOG STRETCHES

- If your knees and wrists will allow, come to all fours on the floor.
- Please use a mat or rug; you may need additional padding under the knees.
- Stack the joints: wrists under shoulders, knees under hips.
- On an inhale, tilt the tailbone up, feel the torso drop down and arch the lower back.
- Open the shoulders, arch the upper back, and then reach up and back with the crown of the head. Be like a tortoise, reaching your head out of its shell.
- On the exhale, start with the tailbone and gently tuck it under, rounding the low and mid-back, then the shoulders.
- Finally tuck your chin so that you look something like a "Halloween cat."
- Reverse back into your dog tilt – follow the inhale.
- Make an effort to start the movement from the tailbone each time.
- Allow the breath to lead your movements. Keep eyes closed or maintain a soft gaze.
- Doing this slowly, vertebrae by vertebrae, will increase your mobility and flexibility over time.

MODIFICATIONS

- Sit back on the heels, hands on thighs, to do these movements on a smaller scale.
- Sit cross-legged or in half-lotus with hands on knees, elevate hips as necessary (sit on a cushion).
- Sit on the edge of a chair seat and rest the hands on the thighs as you move back and forth.
- Try this in a standing position; the movement will be more subtle than when you are sitting or on all fours.

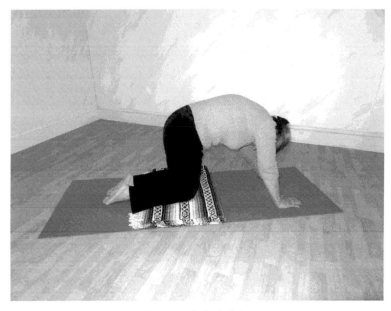

Cat stretch (exhale)

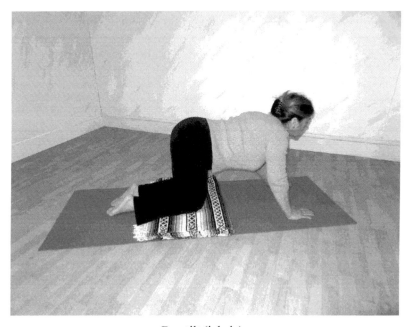

Dog tilt (inhale)

CHAPTER 6: FOCUSING INSIDE

DAY 6

We are accustomed to looking outside of ourselves for most things: love, approval, acceptance, or simply a frame of reference. We compare ourselves to each other and critique ourselves in the mirror. It is constant and never-ending, rooted in that myth that "we are not enough," and it wears us down. We lose our connection to our inner voice and our center when we depend on external forces and other people to judge, help, and fix us. We forget that our true power is really inside us all of the time – we need to be reminded that healing begins on the inside.

There is no way for anyone but you to know how you truly feel and how you might adjust your body or mind to relieve any discomfort. What most of us have forgotten is how to trust and follow our highest, natural instincts. Tuning back into those is an integral part of the holistic healing process.

When we synch up the breath with movement, it helps us to break that dependency on the external world and focus our attention *inside*. We have a chance to shift our attention out of the head and down into the heart and physical body, letting sensation and awareness take over and allowing the brain to rest.

The minute we **stop, slow down, and breathe**, the mind is able to settle; the focus can shift down into sensation as we come in for a landing. If we proceed to gently bring the shoulders back, come into a more "open" body position, and close the eyes, the parasympathetic nervous system will induce the Relaxation Response, which allows the body to rest and re-charge its energy supply. This also allows us to sleep peacefully – a very important ingredient for complete healing.

For this reason, I like to remind my students and clients to close the eyes or use a "soft gaze" while moving in place or holding a pose that is coordinated with the breath. In a soft gaze, you allow the eyes to be slightly open but unfocused, sort of that fuzzy vision we have when we first wakeup in the morning.

When we focus intently on one point, we engage muscles around the eyes and in the face and scalp. Outward focus is not necessary for a majority of the movements or poses in the program; the breath is all you need to focus on, so let your gaze soften, let go of your thoughts. When external stimulation is removed and external light sources are dimmed by closing or unfocusing the eyes, we stimulate the parasympathetic nervous system and the pineal gland. The pineal gland is located in the cranial cavity, behind the forehead. It is responsible for the production and release of melatonin, which regulates our sleep. We'll look at more information on the profound healing we can experience through triggering the parasympathetic nervous system in future chapters.

Even though we live in the 21st century and have made amazing advances in technology, medicine, and science, we need to keep in mind that we are still operating with a DNA configuration from the Stone Age. So how do we adapt Stone Age DNA to a chaotic modern world? Awareness is the foundation needed for changing our responses —and deep breathing opens us up and encourages awareness.

Below are some questions to help you assess some of your blocks and triggers to focusing inside. Complete the following sentences as honestly and accurately as possible. If there is more than one trigger, make a list of all the things that trigger each of these emotional responses. Write down your first thoughts and see if you can become more aware as these feelings kick in, and then choose a different approach next time, using the second list.

I feel afraid when _____.

I feel anxious when _____.

I feel hopeless when _____.

I become depressed when _____.

I feel frustrated when _____.

How can you counteract these feelings and responses in the body? Take a deep breath (or as many as you need) and focus inside. Now let's see what triggers positive responses.

I feel safe when _____.

I feel peaceful when _____.

I feel hopeful when _____.

I feel joyful when _____.

I feel acceptance when _____.

AFFIRMATION: I BREATHE, RELAX, FEEL, WATCH, AND ALLOW, FOCUSING MY ATTENTION INSIDE.

BREATH: ALTERNATE NOSTRIL (NADI SHODHANA)

- Sit comfortably in a chair or on the floor with your spine supported.
- Make sure you sit up tall. Let the shoulders drop down and back, opening the chest. Allow the eyes to be closed.
- Take your right hand and bend down then index and middle fingers.
- Place the right thumb against the right nostril and take a long, slow inhale through the left nostril, filling belly, ribs and finally upper chest.
- Close off the left nostril with your ring finger as you lift the thumb and exhale fully through the right nostril.
- Then take another slow, deep inhale through the right nostril and repeat the pattern.
- This breath balances the sides of the body and the hemispheres of the brain; it calms the central nervous system.
- Take 10 long, slow inhales and 10 long, slow exhales.

POSE: ONE KNEE INTO CHEST

- Come down onto your back and let one knee gently come up towards your chest. The other leg is extended out on the floor. (You may also place the sole of the foot on the floor.)
- If possible, clasp your hands around the knee on top. If this is difficult or at all uncomfortable, use a strap just below the kneecap, or hold onto the thigh in the crease of the knee.
- Relax the head and neck on the floor. There should be no muscle tension in the body.
- Breathe in and out. Feel the extension of the spine on the inhale and the release of the low back and hip as you exhale the knee a bit more into the chest. Please do not force this! Just let the breath move you— you will naturally release when your body is ready.
- Stay for 3-5 breaths.

40

- Gently release the knee and allow the sole of the foot to rest on the floor as you pull the other knee up and in to the chest.

** Use extreme caution on the knee-to-chest move if you have osteoporosis or osteopenia.

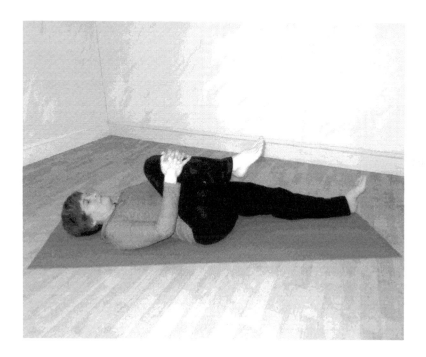

CHAPTER 7: GETTING TO THE ROOT OF YOUR PAIN

DAY 7

Knowing others is intelligence; knowing yourself is true wisdom.

Mastering others is strength; mastering yourself is true power.

--Lao Tzu

Compression on the nerves is the primary cause of pain in the spine. We need to learn as much as we can about what is causing this compression and where the root is. The small, gentle movements and breathing techniques you've begun to use each day will begin to help you understand your body and your pain more thoroughly. It can really help to pinpoint where in your body your pain originates from and what exactly aggravates it – a certain movement, sitting in a comfy chair with no support, walking or standing a certain way or maybe it's from playing a sport, lifting, holding and/or carrying a small child or grocery bags.

Perhaps this started as an annoying backache that appeared from time to time, but always went away with some aspirin or a day's rest. Sometimes you were just too busy to pay attention to it, did not take care of the ache, and just kept pushing through it. You did not listen to your body, until it started screaming at you. And then you *had* to listen because you were stopped in your tracks and immobilized for a time.

The spine is a complicated structure of bones, joints held in place by ligaments and muscles. Typical injuries to the back include sprained ligaments, strained muscles, slipped and/or ruptured discs, and irritated joints; any and all of these may cause compression on one or more nerves. Sometimes it's not a <u>big</u> movement or injury that brings on pain, but the simplest of movements; picking something up from the floor, lifting a child, reaching and leaning forward – that can have painful results. Pain and discomfort in the spine may also be caused by arthritis, poor posture, degenerative disease, psychological stress and/or being overweight. Back pain can also directly result from disease of the internal organs, such as kidney stones, kidney infections or blood clots.

Pain can be seen as a great friend; it is the body's way of sending a signal to the nervous system that says "something's not right here." It's a call for help, a red flag. Without pain, we'd be in big trouble! Unfortunately, many of us were trained as children to "grin and bear it" and as a result we may have developed a high pain threshold. This has played into consumerism, procrastination and our concept of "success": we have all been encouraged to disconnect the brain and the body in order to be more productive, make more money, spend more money and keep up with the Joneses. Unfortunately, if you ignore initial warning signs until the pain is severe, your choices will be significantly diminished and more drastic depending on exactly what's wrong and where.

Remember that living in pain is a choice. You have some other options besides, denial and narcotics, but as you are discovering through this program by now – more effort on your part is required. Chronic pain is tricky because it tends to flare up and die down and after awhile you can get de-sensitized to some of the discomfort and you can fool yourself into thinking that you don't need to keep up your stretching and strengthening program - until it flares up again.

Where you feel the pain may not be its origin.

One of the challenges in Western medicine is the tendency towards isolation: treating the body in parts instead of as a whole – treating the symptoms rather than the cause. That is what allopathic (Western) medicine is all about— pinpointing the disease and focusing solely on eradicating it. This type of medicine is great for trauma, acute conditions and the emergency room, but in the case of chronic conditions, soft tissue injuries, and many spinal injuries and orthopedic issues, it can fail to offer complete healing.

If you don't get to the root of the pain and work on healing beyond the physical, your recovery may be fleeting – pain and symptoms will most likely return and possibly worsen.

See if this sounds familiar: all of the sudden, you wake up one morning with severe lower back pain. You have no history of back injury and no recollection of injuring yourself, but you are barely able to straighten up without experiencing excruciating pain. You can't drive or get to work, so you find someone to take you to your primary physician who tells you to rest, take some Tylenol and use ice or heat, maybe get a massage or see an osteopath (if that's something they value). You try this routine and there is some relief, but very soon the pain is back.

If you keep going back to your Western medical doctor with the same complaint, he or she will most likely order an X-ray and if nothing is seen on the X-ray, physical therapy may be prescribed. This can be very helpful for strengthening the abs and low back, but again, once the therapy is over and you go back to your old habits, you lose the strength and the pain resurfaces.

Now you are worried, scared, uncomfortable, in pain again and feeling vulnerable. If you just can't take the pain any more, you may be sent to an orthopedist and possibly an orthopedic surgeon who will take an MRI of the area. And in the meantime, you get stronger pain medication in order to help you get through each day.

None of these traditional medical approaches are "bad" or "wrong." They are simply incomplete. Very few of your medical practitioners will look at you as a whole being. No one asks you about your lifestyle—your daily habits, your nutrition, your caffeine or alcohol intake, your desk/work station set-up at home or at the office, your car seat, or how you bend down and lift objects. No one has paid attention to your posture or your breathing, which is most likely too shallow. And probably no one has asked about your 20-year-old mattress with the dip in the middle and your 10-year-old pillow which does not support your neck.

Everything in the above paragraph is connected. Everything has a cause and an effect. In the case of acute low back or neck pain, alleviating the pain is necessary and requires localized attention in that area to bring down swelling and reduce pressure on the nerves, but the area that is aggravated is not necessarily where the pain began.

If you can pinpoint the exact cause (and there may be a number of factors involved) not only will this help you heal more completely, but you will also be alert to preventing a similar situation in the future.

In alternative therapies, clients take more of an active role in their own healing; it becomes more of a partnership. And let's face it, there are some people who just don't want to bother. They want someone else to do the work, to wave a magic wand or give them a special pill to fix them quickly and with minimal effort or trouble. You have bought this program, so I think it's safe to assume that you don't belong to that camp.

In the next chapter, we'll get into your lifestyle and habits, but for now, here are some basic questions to consider – you probably already answered some of these in writing the "story" of your low back or neck pain from the introduction:

Is your back pain the result of an injury?

How long have you had the pain?

Did you have any previous history of spinal pain or trauma before this episode?

Is it acute (sharp and shooting) or dull and aching?

AFFIRMATION: BY SIMPLY BREATHING & PAYING ATTENTION TO SENSATION, I AM BECOMING AN EXPERT ON MY OWN BODY AND WHAT IT NEEDS.

POSE/MOVEMENT: BOTH KNEES INTO CHEST

- Bring both knees in towards your chest.
- Gently wrap your hands around them below the kneecaps and keep a gentle pressure.
- Modification: Bend your knees over your hands and hold onto your hamstrings.
- Let yourself rock & roll gently, from side to side, massaging the lumbar spine area.
- **** Do NOT do the Double Knee into Chest move if you have osteoporosis or osteopenia. Repeat the One Knee into Chest (from yesterday), with caution.**

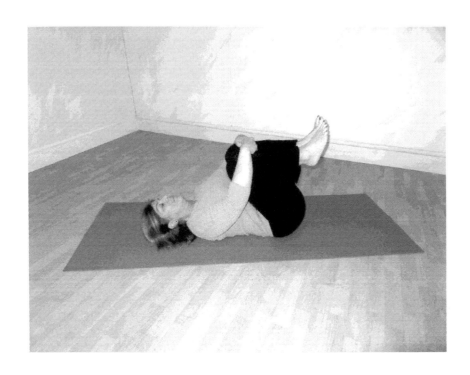

CHAPTER 8: DEALING WITH OVERSTIMULATION

DAY 8

We can control the thoughts we have in our heads and how we move our bodies. We can also control what we eat and drink and look at; the conversations we participate in, the people we socialize with, etc. Each of these elements play a powerful part in changing your physiology and well-being. Even though there are many ways to be overwhelmed by the external world, lifestyle management and nutrition may prove to be two of the most effective and easily accessible antidotes to stress and overstimulation.

Ayurveda, the sister science to yoga, is a form of self-healing and lifestyle management that has been practiced for more than 5,000 years. Ayurveda instructs us in how to live in harmony with nature and within our own bodies. It addresses everything from physical, mental, emotional and spiritual issues to our eating and sleeping habits. Its basic premise is that all health and disease begin in the digestive tract and that we must maintain a proper amount of digestive fire (agni) in order for optimal health.

Therapeutic yoga, breathing techniques and meditation practices are frequently recommended for many conditions and ailments. Try bringing awareness to the following aspects of your life and looking at how they affect your feelings of overstimulation and anxiety.

Caffeine intake

If you drink caffeinated coffee, tea, sodas, energy drinks, and/or eat chocolate (even the "good" dark chocolate) you need to be aware of the effects these stimulants have on your body.

All foods and beverages with caffeine create the physiological stress responses that lower metabolism and store fat. Once in a while, this is okay, but constant overstimulation leads to the feeling of burnout – because the adrenals are firing off their hormones constantly and our systems can overload.

Look at your caffeine intake alongside your lifestyle habits and you might see a connection and how they affect one another. You get tired, so you need a "pick-me-up" at work—a Coke, a cup of coffee, a sugary snack or piece of chocolate. And what does this do? It stimulates the adrenal glands even more and though that may seem like a good thing at first, most of us have discovered that after the rush, we crash again. When the adrenals are stressed, they produce cortisol and adrenaline which are released into the bloodstream to help cope with the effects of stress. Ultimately this cycle contributes to overtaxing the adrenal glands and wearing them out (see Chapter 11).

If your body is in this constant state of exhaustion and you are a regular coffee, black tea, caffeinated soda drinker, or chocolate-eater, the best antidote is to cut down on or stop your caffeine intake entirely. I know people get very defensive around their coffee habits in particular, so perhaps you can treat this as an experiment. Try to cut back to one cup of coffee in the morning. If you are already at that place, then try a cup of coffee every other day.

Switching to decaffeinated coffee or tea is always an alternative —you get the same taste without the stimulation, but beware: decaf coffee actually is much more acidic than regular. While we all need a healthy "digestive fire" in our stomach and intestines to breakdown food, acidic foods and beverages (like alcohol) create excess fire in the gut. This creates an imbalance of "pitta" dosha in Ayurveda, which can lead to ulcers and more serious digestive disorders. Too much acid in the system also dehydrates your tissues and organs.

They now have special "alkaline drops" you can purchase online to add to your coffee (or any highly acidic beverage, including your drinking water) – these change the pH, neutralizing the acid and thereby making it more alkaline and less harsh on your stomach and intestines.

Make changes slowly and make notes in your Healing Journal on how you feel -- notice any effects that manifest in the body or mind.

Food and Beverage Temperature

Ayurveda focuses on calming and/or stoking the digestive fire in order to aid in the breakdown of food and absorption of the nutrients. You've stimulated those digestive enzymes the minute food is placed in the mouth; the stomach gets ready to release acid – you are preparing your fire. When the fire is doused and food is in the stomach, it sits there. This can lead to gas, bloating and eventually more serious digestive issues and diseases.

We don't have any other way to breakdown our food except with this fire of acid and enzymes. Our stomach reacts by releasing more acid – it has no choice. And we end up with heartburn, indigestion, acid reflux… and, in desperation, reach for a Rolaids or a Tums. The antacid business wouldn't exist without those ice cold drinks

The irony is, if you just changed some of your eating and drinking habits and the foods and beverages you are consuming, you wouldn't have the problem, wouldn't feel this discomfort and wouldn't need the pills. Taking sips of room temperature or warm water or other gut-friendly beverages are an easy shift to make. Certain herbal teas or a cup of hot water can be very healing to the digestive tract.

Do your best to drink your larger amounts of fluids in between meals, on an empty stomach. And when you drink with your meals, just take little sips in between food – so that you don't flood the stomach and wash out all of the enzymes and naturally occurring acid.

As far as food temperature goes, there is a similar correlation: cold foods contribute to stagnation and constipation. Warm/hot foods are more easily digested. I don't mean "hot and spicy" foods, but the temperature of the food itself. Also, please take into consideration seasonal changes as well as your geographical climate and weather – on a sweltering hot summer day, some cool beverages and/or raw foods tend to be more tolerable and appropriate.

Smoking

Smoking inhibits the absorption of oxygen by the lungs and disrupts normal blood flow in the body. Blood flow is how oxygen and nutrients get to the brain and all vital organs of the body, the spine, the muscles, etc. This is a deadly habit. We've known it for years now. Quit smoking! You are slowly suffocating yourself -- it's as simple as that.

They now have the electronic and vapor cigarettes available to help you quit smoking regular cigarettes. I don't know how effective these are compared to the nicotine patches and acupuncture treatments, but look into all of your options.

The body is your temple, keep it pure and clean for the soul to reside in.

-B.K.S. Iyengar

Refined carbohydrates

Refined carbohydrates such as white sugar, white flour, white bread, and high fructose corn syrup turn to glucose in the blood. The presence of excess glucose in the blood triggers the pancreas to create more insulin. Insulin causes the liver, skeletal muscles, and fat tissue to take up glucose from the blood.

If you are eating many simple carbohydrates a few times a day, every day, your body is working overtime releasing insulin to break them down. Many years of this overuse of the pancreas can lead to diabetes. If you have a family history of diabetes or your system tends to be sensitive in other ways, this disease may have an early onset when you are quite young.

Refined carbs give a rush to your system. If you consume them regularly and/or in large quantities, the constant high levels of glucose will stimulate repeated releases of insulin. This causes the cells to become resistant to insulin binding to the membranes and makes it harder for the cells to absorb the glucose. As a result, the levels of glucose in the blood rise, making it more toxic. The cells then starve for energy and this drop in cellular energy is why you feel brain and body fatigue and why you crave more carbs, and how you can get into the vicious cycle of sugar highs and sugar crashes.

Any time a food is "refined" that means that it has been heated to an extremely high temperature. Initially, this was used primarily for food safety and purification – to kill bacteria. Unfortunately, the process of refining, literally "burns out" most of the nutrients that our bodies really need and leaves us the leftovers which are harder for our systems to digest. Refined products can be produced and sold in mass quantities and they have a long shelf life. This is just one way in which "convenience" undoes us, over and over again. Cut back on your consumption of these processed and refined items and see if you notice a difference. Write down observations in your journal.

High Fructose corn syrup is the "new sugar" and the biggest culprit in the alarming rise of juvenile obesity and diabetes in this country. It's much easier and cheaper to produce high fructose corn syrup than it is to grow and harvest sugar cane and process it.

Genetically modified organisms (GMOs) are something to be aware of regarding any corn consumption – read your labels and decide if you really want to eat foods that are grown from "pest-resistant seeds." In plain English that means that the pesticide has been inserted into the DNA of the seed. No one really knows what the long-term effects of this consumption will be, but my personal feeling is that people should not be the guinea pigs. Also, an interesting and startling fact is that these GMO seeds can only be used once; the plants they produce are sterile, meaning their seeds are no good. All of the farmers using this seed have to buy more each year since they are no longer able to save and using the natural seeds from last season's crop.

Go through your kitchen cabinets and start reading the labels on all the processed foods you have. Get rid of what you can afford to, especially if it has lots of long chemical compounds listed that you can't pronounce. The best approach to an overall healthy diet is to stick to whole, unprocessed, natural, fresh foods (usually these are complex carbohydrates) —the less packaging, the better. This is part of your awareness training.

Media overload

Whenever I think of media overload, I think of the famous scene in "Network," a great film from the 70's, where Peter Finch's character encourages everyone to open their windows and yell the line "I'm mad as hell and I'm not going to take this anymore." And in the film, television sets are seen being hurled out of windows. While I don't think it's necessary to smash your TV to the ground, I do think it makes sense to "take back" those evenings and weekends that get lost on a regular basis in re-runs and reality shows. Everything in moderation.

The media is a powerful stimulant, much more so than in the 70's. Everywhere we turn these days, we are bombarded by advertisements and way too much information in print, talk, and video. They even post print ads on the stall doors of public restrooms now; whole buses are colorful ads on wheels and perhaps you've experienced the advertisements printed on the floors of New York City subway stations. So even if you try to look down, away from walls and billboards, you still can't escape—they're under your feet as well.

Have you noticed how television commercials have also gotten **louder**? This is another little trick that advertisers have come up with to get your attention: They increase the volume, making the commercials quite a bit louder than the program you're watching. This is especially true during sports programs. There was a law passed to regulate this, but I don't know if it is being enforced with any regularity. I have not noticed any improvement with shows I have watched. In any case, keep your finger ready on the mute button when you do watch any TV.

During these 30 days, experiment with limiting your television intake. If you want to go cold turkey, that's great. If that's too drastic a commitment, then try a significant cutback and make notes on how it affects you and your stress levels. Use your mute button generously.

Cell phones and Internet

Internet and e-mail can also over-stimulate your mind and your whole physiology—your eyes and mind take in all the ads, news, and other information that you're bombarded with but all systems are affected. E-mail, as I can personally attest to, can turn into an addiction. Yes, it's communication, but it's disconnected communication, and we want to focus on connecting mind and body as much as possible.

Whether we're talking about media, work, or home life, that feeling that we are not quite enough and always need to "keep up with the Joneses" is completely draining on a daily basis. The more you limit the external stimulation around you, the more energy you will have to focus on your healing and catch up on sleeping and interacting with your partner, kids, friends, and family.

Try turning off your cell phone whenever you don't <u>absolutely</u> need to be reached for work or emergencies. For many years we all did just fine without these devices—maybe business was conducted at a slower pace, but it was more civilized and no one was tethered to an electronic device wherever they were outside of the workplace.

Be smarter than your smart phone: give the texting and tweeting a rest. Do your absolute best to cut back or go cold turkey for the rest of your time with this program so that you become more familiar with your own pace and rhythm of life instead of letting outside, technical forces dictate this for you. If you could pinpoint this as the antidote to total healing and a pain-free life, wouldn't you do it? Think of this as part of your experiment and see what happens.

Intense people and relationships

We all know that difficult co-workers, bosses, family members and in-laws can cause us a great deal of stress, but similarly, you may have friends who mean well, but who take up a lot of your time and energy with their drama. I'm sure you've experienced this at one time or another, or maybe someone in your life qualifies right now. Julia Cameron, author of *The Artist's Way*, calls these people "crazy makers"; their lives are out of control, they seem to be in a constant state of panic or emergency. They have a desperate need to dump all of their worries and issues on those around them who will listen. These people can add to your stress and distract you from your own self-care. They are <u>not</u> helping you to heal. You can send them loving, compassionate energy, but you don't need these energetic vampires around you.

Try to remove yourself from these people and their drama as much as possible; see if you can distance yourself for the rest of the program at least. If he or she is a family member for whom you are a caregiver, see if another relative or friend can help out. Get creative in your thinking – ask for help. This is how you can protect your own energy and your healing process.

Nine times out of ten, this is one of the big "missing pieces" to the healing puzzle. Our relationships and interactions with others need to be loving and supportive, not toxic and draining. If you choose to love yourself enough to create and enforce healthy boundaries around your time and space, this could end up being one of your best "painkillers"! And your willingness to try this may be a main component of complete healing for your chronic condition.

The charts on the next few pages will help you get a more complete picture of how you are running your life and/or how your life is running you. Once you can see this clearly, the plan you can use to shift is pretty simple – do the opposite for a very different, life-changing set of results.

Yesterday I was clever, so I wanted to change the world.
Today I am wise, so I am changing myself.
-Rumi

We either make ourselves miserable or make ourselves strong,
but the amount of work is the same.
-Carlos Castaneda

Nutrition/Nourishment Assessment

Question	Answer (yes or no)	If yes, how many times per day & how much?
I drink caffeinated coffee.		
I drink other caffeinated beverages (soda, energy drinks, tea).		
I eat chocolate (milk or dark).		
I eat refined carbs (white sugar and flour).		
I drink alcohol.		
I use ice in my drinks and everything comes out of the fridge.		
I eats fruits and vegetables on a daily basis.		
I drink purified water on a regular basis.		
I eat meat (steak, chicken, fish?)		
I eat sitting down at the table with my family or housemates.		
I eat slowly and mindfully.		
I eat my biggest meal of the day between 12noon and 2pm.		
I eat after 8pm at night.		
I eat my meals at the same times each day.		

Nutrition/Nourishment Targets

Ideal: STOP drinking the coffee, the sodas and the alcohol consumption all together. Helpful: Cut back and notice the difference.

Coffee substitutes and antidotes: herbal teas, Yerba Mate. Even diluted black tea with some stevia and milk would be better. Even though milk contains lactic acid, it does dilute the affects of coffee's acidity. I mentioned earlier that there are now Alkaline drops available for coffee (or any beverage) to neutralize the acid content.

If you are not willing to give up coffee, at least cut back and keep track of the effects you feel – this may give you further incentive to give it up all together. Note: you probably will have some unpleasant withdrawal symptoms for a period of about 2 to 4 weeks. The main complaints are usually headaches and irritability and agitation; noise level, taste and smell sensitivities. It's all temporary as your body and mind recover and reorganize and well worth the clarity and health benefits on the other side.

The tannins in tea do have health benefits – they are an astringent and a diuretic. Some believe that milk destroys all of the health benefits of the tannins or herbs, while others believe that a little bit of milk reduces the caffeine and dilutes acidity. Ginger tea and green tea are said to be the lowest in acidity.

Sodas/carbonated beverages: Think of the bubbles in a carbonated drink – they fizz up and this same agitation is what you will bring in to your digestive tract. Sodas bring way too much air (vata) into the system – they will create gas, constipation and over time, there is research to confirm that they contribute to bone loss, particularly in women and particularly the cola-based sodas.

Again, if you're not ready and willing to give up soda, at least cut back significantly and keep track of any changes you see and feel. Unless you have a bad chocolate habit, you can probably still have a small piece every now and then – dark chocolate being the healthier alternative.

Cold vs. Room Temperature drinks: Antidote: choose room temperature or warm beverages instead.

Time of eating and amount of food consumed: Eat your biggest meal at the middle of the day when the sun is at its height – more fire on the outside can support your inner digestive fire as well. Do not eat a meal or snack after 8:00pm so that you will be able to fall asleep more easily, without food in your stomach. Digestion takes a lot of energy!

Lifestyle/Habits at Home Assessment

Question	Answer (yes or no)	If yes, how or how often?
I have trouble getting to sleep.		
I have trouble staying asleep.		
I sleep with a bolster or pillow under my knees.		
I sit in bed and read or watch TV.		
I have a favorite comfy chair that I sit in.		
I smoke.		
I have a cardio exercise program that I do.		
I have a strength training program that I do.		
I have neck pain as well as back pain.		
I am always in a rush and never seem to have enough time to get things done.		
I am under stress at home.		
I am not happy in my relationship with my partner.		

The chapters on sleep and ergonomics will help you with the first few questions. Sometimes, just noticing and observing your habits and choices will be enough information for you. We do so many things on auto-pilot and then repeat the routines for years that sometimes we're not even aware of what we're doing or how detrimental it might end up being to ourselves.

Please quit smoking if you haven't yet. Do whatever it takes and you won't regret it -- this will add years to your life and be able to take much deeper, healing breaths. Get some daily exercise of some sort – 20 minutes of walking is great. Gentle yoga is wonderful or perhaps Tai Chi. Use a simple breath meditation for 5 minutes in the morning when you get up and at night before you go to bed, to get out of your head and back in to your body. You can also take a few minutes on your lunch break or any other time during the day to breathe deeply and connect to your center.

Lifestyle/Habits at Work Assessment

Question	Answer (yes or no)	If yes, please elaborate.
I am under a great deal of stress at work.		
I tend to eat whatever is left out in the employee break room.		
I get sugar cravings and then crashes.		
I sit or stand for most of the day without a break.		
I work more than 10 hours per day.		
I do repetitive, manual labor or repetitive, mental work -- reading, typing.		
I have ergonomic props for my desk & computer and I use them.		
I answer phones frequently and use a headset.		
I am able to get away from my desk at lunch and take a walk.		
I bring my lunch and it's usually something healthy.		
I forget to eat when I am under a deadline.		
I drink water at work. (cold or room temp)		
Ladies – I wear high heels at work on a regular basis.		

The best antidote to some of these lifestyle work habits that are not healthy is to adopt a more serious meditation practice. It will connect you to your true essence, remind you that you are so much more than your job and your tasks, and again, slow you down. You may say "I can't slow down – I have so much to get done!" And that right there is exactly why you need to slow down – if you don't, you will burn yourself and your adrenal glands out and your spinal issues will get worse. Ironically, you will find that if you slow down and become more mindful about everything you do – work and play – you will actually be more productive in your life and in the world. The rushing around that we do comes from a deep fear of scarcity – that there's not enough to go around, and that we're not enough. And both of these things could not be more false.

Most of the other antidotes are intuitive: it's good to take breaks from your work; you need to feed and nourish your body with healthy foods and to drink enough water to stay hydrated. Skip the junk food and get off of the high heels for added benefits to your overall well-being.

Lifestyle/Habits in the Car Assessment

Question	Yes or No	Please elaborate.
I commute by car more than 30 minutes each way to work.		
I carpool.		
I have some sort of back support cushion.		
I always hold the top of the wheel.		
I frequently get stuck in traffic.		
Traffic stresses me out and I get angry at the other drivers.		
I listen to music or books on CD and make the most of my time in the car.		
My hips and low back are killing me when I get out of the car.		
I commute by bus or train more than 30 minutes each way.		
I listen to music or books on CD and make the most of my time in the bus or train.		

If you have a long commute to and from your workplace, get an ergonomic evaluation of you in your car – it helps to have someone else look at your positioning and your car seat, where your elbows fall and whether or not your spine rounds and you lead with your chin, with the head pulled forward in front of the rest of the body. All of these things can be remedied with props or other tools.

One universal tip that is helpful: notice if you grip the top of the steering wheel with your hands as you drive and what effect this has on your shoulders and neck. Try a simple adjustment – bring the hands down and out to 4pm and 8pm on the wheel if you are looking at it like a clock. Notice how your shoulders release and so does the neck. Let yourself get used to driving in this position.

If you do find you get incredibly stressed in traffic, soft jazz or classical music can be a soothing soundtrack in the background or listen to an audio book. You can also use your breath meditation, with open eyes of course, and not Nadi Shodhana which requires you to use your hands. Simply breathe in and out and imagine you are filling up and emptying out a balloon.

Also, while safely at a stop or pulled over to the side of the road, you can do your Cat and Dog motions (p.39-40) with the breath and Side to Side lateral movements in your seat, and even a gentle twist – the range of motion may not be great, but it will stretch out the neck, low back and hips.

More antidotes

You can't control the stressful situations and people around you, but you can remove yourself from their presence in the short term. And long-term, there are things you can do to alleviate the effects of stress on your body and mind.

Rest: Getting enough rest helps to balance the effects of stress. Studies show that stress plays a significant role in weight gain and insomnia. Rest is also essential for allowing the body to rejuvenate naturally. It also can aid in pain management and relief (more on this in Chapter 22 and 23.).

Environment: You deserve a special space, a safe environment in which to read this book, do your movements, go over affirmations and write in your journal. If you haven't already done so, create a space in your house which will be used solely for the purposes of your healing. It may just be an uncluttered corner of a room, a special sitting area—there is no right or wrong way for it to look -- make it warm and inviting.

If you live with a partner, roommate, and/or kids, set some boundaries around this area; let them know that it is off-limits to them and consider giving them a schedule of when you will be using the space and going through your practice. Don't let anyone or anything disturb you while you are in this space—it's your safety zone. If you value and respect yourself and your healing process and emphasize the importance of it to others, they will listen and respect you. That also creates another kind of healing—communicating: being heard and seen and hearing and seeing others.

For more support with lifestyle evaluations, please consult an Ayurvedic health consultant. I offer telephone or Skype consultations to those who live too far away for an in-person appointment.

AFFIRMATION: I MAKE HEALTHY, CONSCIOUS CHOICES IN EACH MOMENT WHICH CULTIVATE HEALING ENERGY.

MOVEMENT: HAMSTRING STRETCH WITH STRAP

- Lie on the floor on your back with knees bent.
- Take a strap, belt, or tie and wrap it around both feet.
- Push your feet up towards the ceiling. Point your heels up and toes down.
- Inhale and on the exhale give a gentle tug on the strap, pulling your legs toward you.
- Don't force the stretch; breathe into it. Back off if it gets too intense.
- Stay for 2 to 3 breaths each time. Do this 3 times.

- You can also do this one leg at a time, using your other foot on the ground for support – see photos on next page.

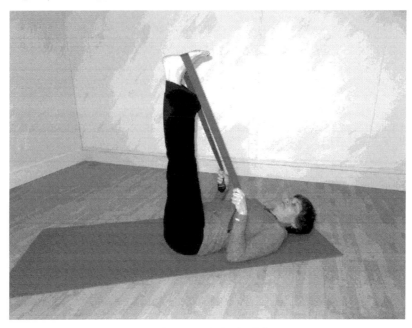

Hamstring stretch for both legs

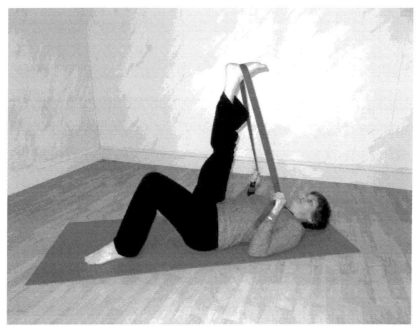

Hamstring stretch with strap (each leg)

CHAPTER 9: CRASH COURSE IN SPINAL ANATOMY

DAY 9

You may have seen an X-ray of your spine at some point, but these high-light the bony structure only – the vertebrae and ribs. I see this as one of the downfalls of western medicine – it takes such an in-depth, specific view of one area of our physical bodies when we are sick, often at the expense of the other systems that are connected to the area where the trouble reveals itself. In order to heal completely, it's necessary to get to know the nuts and bolts of your body and how it all works together – how the muscles, tendons and ligaments serve to hold the vertebrae in place and support the discs as well.

Getting to Know Your Spine

The spinal cord is housed in the protective bony structure know as the vertebral or spinal column. The bony spine is comprised of **33 vertebrae:**

7 cervical vertebrae (the neck area), 12 thoracic vertebrae (upper and middle back), 5 lumbar vertebrae (low back), 5 vertebrae that are naturally fused together to form the sacrum, and 4 vertebrae that form the tailbone. The non-fused vertebrae are each separated by an **intervertebral disc**.

The discs serve as "cushions," absorbing the shock of your movements. Think of your discs as jelly donuts—a gel-like substance in the middle surrounded by a tougher fibrocartilaginous (fiber and cartilage) structure. Discs are meant to "give" and move, but only so much. They not only absorb vibrations, but their cushioning also protects your nerves. Each vertebra has a couple of holes on either side through which the nerves thread and span out into the body.

The collagen in the discs is affected by the loss of water content; disc height can also be lost as they weaken and wear out, as fluids become depleted, leading to bulging and herniation. As we age, our bodies dry out, so part of this loss is natural and can be expected. This loss of height is happening to many people at a younger age and is a direct result of poor lifestyle and nutrition choices, poor ergonomics and body mechanics, stress. It is a slow, degenerative process that may be happening regardless of injury.

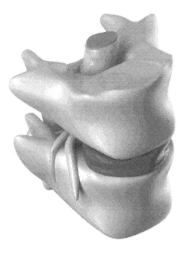

Spinal cord with nerves branching out

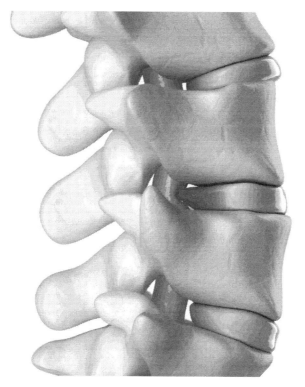

Protrusion: Bulging disc compressing nerve

When the jelly part of the disc or "donut" has literally been squeezed too far forward or backward between the vertebrae, the disc **bulges**, which pushes on the nerves. If the jelly moves further out of the disc this is called a **protrusion**. When the part of the jelly has moved completely out of the donut, and is actually dripping, with part of it torn off on the outside, this is a **herniated disc.**

As this process progresses, the torn piece of the disc moves away from the immediate area **(prolapse)**, the vertebrae end up closer together, further compressing nerves. If the herniation gets worse, all of the gel could be squeezed out of the middle of your disc, leaving you with bone rubbing on bone which is very painful. This leads to the degeneration of the facet joints.

In an effort to repair itself, the spine will form bone spurs. Then the joints enlarge (causing **osteoarthritis**, or **degenerative disc disease**) and this causes the spinal ligaments to thicken and lose their strength and elasticity. Ultimately, it is the bone spurs that cause the most nerve compression, but any decrease in disc height shifts the alignment of the spine and can cause discomfort or pain that sometimes shoots into other areas of the body. Most commonly, pain shoots down the legs when the sciatic nerve is being compressed.

The purpose of the vertebral column is two-fold: 1) to protect the spinal cord, which runs the length of the spine, with nerves branching out into the various extremities, and 2) to allow flexion and extension of the trunk of the body from an upright position, to protect the brain, spinal cord, and nerves by absorbing shock.

The vertebral discs are not meant to move very much, but flexion (forward bends) and extension (back bends) are healthy movements for the trunk. Side-to-side and gentle twisting are also good and necessary movements for the spine (we'll discuss these movements further in Chapter 12) and can be even safer if you remember to breathe with the movement. The breath will create the space—the extra bit of extension needed in the spine —to move safely without wearing down and injuring the discs.

The good news: The vertebral column is supported and held in place by an intricate muscular system. More good news: structural issues and misalignment in the spine are usually due to weak or strained muscles. This can be remedied. We can always strengthen, stretch or rest and heal the soft tissue around the bones to correct the misalignment.

Be not afraid of growing slowly;
be afraid only of standing still.
-Chinese Proverb

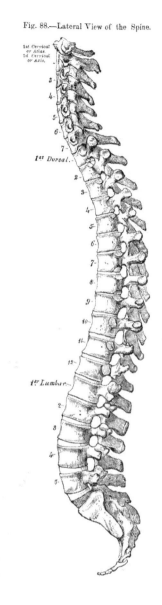

Fig. 88.—Lateral View of the Spine.

AFFIRMATION: KNOWLEDGE IS POWER AND I ENJOY LEARNING MORE ABOUT MY BODY AND HOW IT WORKS.

MOVEMENT: HIP OPENERS

- Using a yoga strap, a bathrobe belt, or a couple of men's ties tied together (get creative!), lie on your back, bring your knees into your chest, and wrap the strap around the right foot.
- Push the foot in the strap up towards the ceiling and leave the other leg on the ground (you can bend the knee for the first part of this).
- Slowly allow the leg in the strap to open all the way out to the side until your elbow is anchoring you and it feels like your foot is hanging in the "sling" created by the strap.
- Stretch your left arm out to the side and rest it on the floor.
- Take deep breaths as you hold here. If you have any pain or discomfort, give yourself more slack with the strap. See if you are able to keep your leg straight.
- Do this for approximately 1-2 minutes and inhale your right leg back up over center, extend the other leg out (if knee was bent) and switch hands with the strap.
- Slowly let the leg come across your body and over to the left side. The hip lifts off the floor but the opposite shoulder stays on the floor.
- Allow the elbow to anchor you again. Hopefully you can feel this stretch in the glutes and low back. Breathe deeply in and out.
- Inhale and pull your foot back up over you and lower your leg to the ground slowly and let go of the strap.
- Take a moment on your back, focusing on the breath, and notice if the hip/low back on this side feels any different than the other side.
- Change legs and do the same on the other side. End on your back, breathing in and out. Notice if your hips have balanced out.
- This will still feel great for loosening the hips even if your main problem is in the neck – just make sure you keep the shoulders as relaxed as possible as you hold the strap; give yourself a lot of slack, literally.

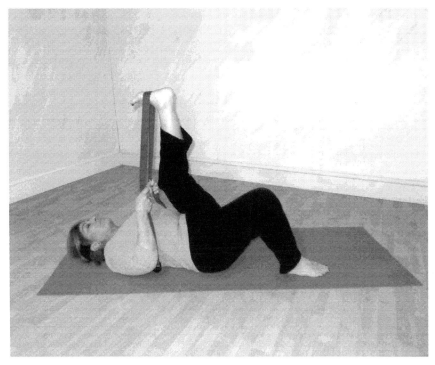

Hip openers (begin with one leg in strap)

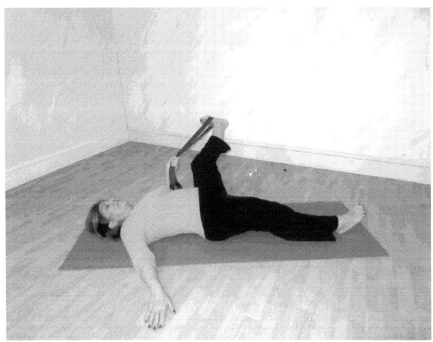

Leg reaches out to one side, opposite arm and shoulder ground you.

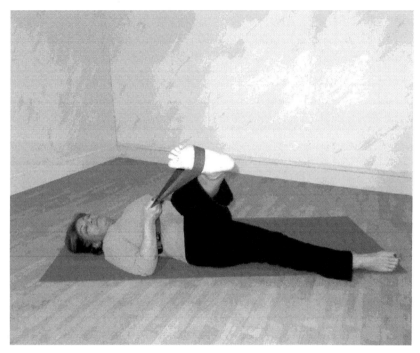

The leg comes all the way over to the other side.

CHAPTER 10: YOUR MUSCULAR SYSTEM

DAY 10

Muscles

Muscle is a very special tissue that is responsible for exerting force and causing motion in the body. Muscle functions and abilities differ according to where they attach and insert in the body. The spine is held in place by an intricately woven system of muscles generally referred to as the "erector spinae." These are the muscles which allow us to stand tall and sit up straight.

The **erector spinae** are in turn covered and supported by layers of larger muscles, such as those in the upper and mid-back like the **rhomboids**, which hold the shoulder blades in place and facilitate movement, and the **trapezius**, which connect at the shoulder girdle and wrap around to the collarbone in front.

In the lower back, the **quadratus lumborum** ("QL" for short) and the **psoas major** help to stabilize the lower spine and when over-tight can cause low back problems. The QL attaches the posterior lower spine to the crest of the hip-bone.

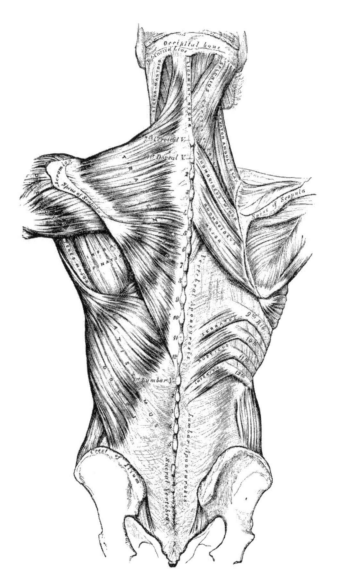

Muscles connecting to the vertebral column

The psoas connects the front of the lumbar spine to the **femur** or thigh bone. Another muscle layer supporting the erectors would be the **serratus posterior**, and covering that is the largest muscle in the body, the **latissimus dorsi**, which stretches across most of the posterior trunk. There are many other important muscles contributing to the healthy movement and stability of the spine, but these are the main ones that will give you a good overview to start. There are many online resources and books that go into great depth on the muscles of the back (see my Resources section).

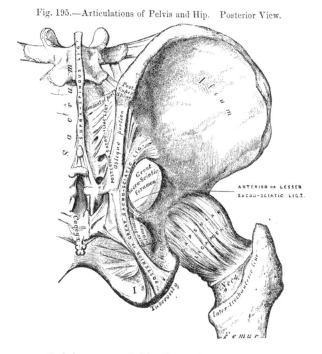

Pelvis, sacrum & hip (front view) with ligaments

The other important muscle that needs mentioning here is also part of the respiratory system: the **diaphragm**. This is a thin, half-dome-shaped muscle that separates the thoracic abdominal cavities. When we inhale, the lungs expand and the diaphragm pushes down on the abdominal organs. As we exhale the breath out, the diaphragm relaxes, rising back up and helping to push the air out of the lungs.

The **intercostal muscles** in between each of the ribs allow the chest to expand and the ribcage to open and rise up.

Tendons link muscle to bone, serving as transmitters of the force created by the muscles. They are responsible for the movement of the joints.

Ligaments are connective tissue that attach one bone to another at the joint. They stabilize the joint, but also allow for a certain degree of mobility. Depending on the function they serve, ligaments can come in all shapes and sizes and usually have some elasticity. The most important thing to remember about ligaments is that they can be easily overstretched and strained. They can also become too tight, which happens frequently in the hip joint, limiting extension: the thinner the ligament, the more mobility in the joint (e.g., the shoulder); the thicker the ligament, the more stability in the joint (e.g., large bony structures like the pelvis and hip joints).

Both tendons and ligaments contain networks of sensory nerves that send messages to the brain regarding muscle tension and joint position.

Good news: If we gently strengthen and stretch the muscles in the spine, the alignment of the vertebrae will adjust and come back into balance.

AFFIRMATION: EVERY DAY I BECOME STRONGER AND MORE FLEXIBLE.

MOVEMENT: HALF LOCUST ON EACH SIDE

- Gather any props you may need to be comfortable on your belly (blankets, pillows, cushions).
- Slowly work your way down onto the floor. Lie face down, resting the forehead on the backs of your hands.
- Feel the legs rest in a hip-width position.
- Inhale, fill the belly, and feel it push against the ground.
- Exhale and engage the abs, feeling the pubic bone push into the ground.

- With the next inhale, reach back with your right toes and, engaging the leg muscles, lift the right leg up.
- Exhale and release the leg down slowly, with control.
- Repeat on the other side and go back and forth for 10 times on each side.
- Allow the floor to stabilize and support you as you do this movement.
- This is great for strengthening the abs and low back.

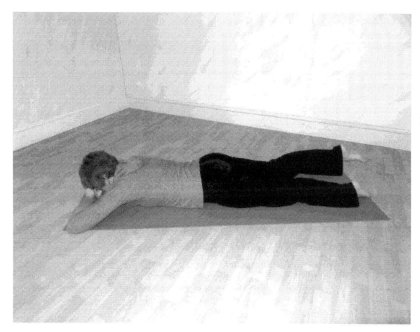

Half Locust – one leg lifted

CHAPTER 11: YOUR CENTRAL NERVOUS SYSTEM

DAY 11

Your brain and your spinal cord make up your central nervous system. The brain is very much like a computer and the spinal cord and peripheral nervous system is its network which relays messages back and forth, via the nerve endings. The nerves transmit messages all the way out to the extremities and back to the brain at lightning speed. Touch a hot stove and the nerves in your fingers send a "pain" signal to the brain. The brain quickly sends a message back to pull the hand away from the stove. Tiny cells called neurons are actually responsible for the transmission of messages through a complicated electrochemical process.

The Sympathetic Nervous System

The sympathetic nervous system (SNS) is considered "autonomic," meaning that it is able to operate without conscious thought, prepping the body for instant action. This system is responsible for triggering our "fight-or-flight response," which acts directly on the cardiovascular system, pumping us up in order to protect ourselves from danger. This is the state that we've come to know as "stress."

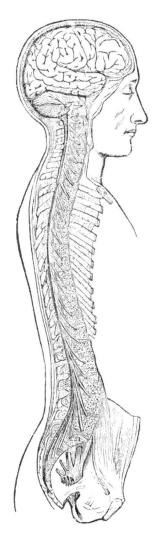

Brain and Spinal Cord – Side View

Back in the days of ferocious dinosaurs and saber-toothed tigers, we needed our fight-or-flight response to flood our systems with **adrenaline** and

cortisol (see Appendix so that we could run fast and escape the danger and survive. We still need this ability at times, when the danger is real, but our poor posture and body positioning can accidentally trigger this response, and if we constantly sit in a hunched over position as if you are protecting yourself, your breathing will naturally be shallow because your chest sinks in, and your central nervous system will interprets these signs to mean that you are in danger.

The Stress Response does not discriminate. Whether you work at a desk or on an assembly line, behind the wheel of a bus or a Mac truck, or out in a field, you have deadlines to meet, tough bosses and difficult co-workers to deal with, white collar, blue collar, doctor, nurse or stay at home mom, if you are hunched over, the message to the brain is the same: your sympathetic nervous system takes our closed body language and shallow breath to mean "danger" and fires off adrenaline and cortisol _all day long_ (or as long as we remain in this position).

This over-stimulates the adrenal glands and exhausts our whole body; ironically, it can also cause sleeping difficulties because our bodies are flooded with these "danger" hormones, with no way to release them from the system and then we feel too tired to get ourselves moving again. As a result we desperately need those cups of coffee and/or afternoon Diet Coke™ to keep us going—and there you have the vicious chain of reaction in which many of us get caught.

If you need to run or perform some other emergency action, "fight or flight" always comes in handy, but keeping ourselves in a constant state of panic is simply not a healthy way to live. It causes many complications over a prolonged period of time and prevents us from connecting our breath and bodies, and keeps us distracted and thus open to injury and accidents.

No problem can be solved from the same level
of consciousness that created it.
-Albert Einstein

The Parasympathetic Nervous System

The parasympathetic nervous system (PSNS) counters and yet complements the sympathetic system. The PSNS kicks in when we draw back our shoulders, open our chest cavity, sit up straight, and take full, deep breaths. It is also engaged when the eyes are unfocused and/or closed, blocking out the stimulating effects of light. Relaxing hormones are released when this system takes over, and deep healing can occur. The average Westerner's body is in dire need of relaxation and unwinding, but we must feel safe before we can rest soundly.

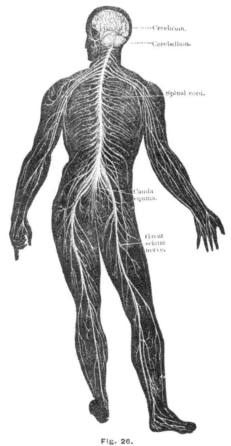

Fig. 26.
General Representation of the Nervous System.

Pain Relief Recipe: Shifting into Neutral

This whole program offers you many different ingredients that can be used together to relieve chronic, and many times acute, pain. I thought I would be helpful to outline the whole philosophy I have around how this unfolds. Much of it is simply knowing how the nervous system functions and reacts – how it responds to pain and how the rest of the body's systems go into action and protection mode once the pain message is received. And we each have our own unique experiences of this.

When the eyes are open and the brain is in gear, the wheels are turning and we are propelled forward by our thoughts. When in gear, our brain can and will enable us to go "faster", to multi-task, etc., but that's not always necessary and it's sometimes detrimental. A good example would be one of those sleepless nights when our body is quite tired, but our mind is racing in high gear and we just can't seem to shut it off and so we are not able to rest because we can't shift into neutral.

In order to relieve any pain in our body and begin to heal on a deep and permanent level, we need to shift the whole body-mind-spirit into "neutral", starting with the Central Nervous System. Luckily, any type of therapeutic yoga and breathing exercise can accomplish this. With each day and each chapter, I hope you are beginning to really see and experience more wholeness within you as you expand your awareness and feel yourself healing in a whole new way. As you allow yourself to go deeper inside with this process, you can also step back further in order to get more perspective.

Closing your eyes is the first step. This stops the onslaught of visual information coming in to the brain. The muscles around the eyes and in the face can all relax when the eyes close. You can close your eyes in any of the poses and movements introduced so far.

Remember that taking deep deliberate breaths and using techniques to focus our attention in a meditation is another major ingredient of the recipe. This allows more oxygen into the bloodstream and improves your circulation. The expanded lungs massage your heart at the same time.

Lying down on a firm, supportive surface with props as needed under head and knees is also instrumental in relieving compression on the nerves. A mat or blanket on the floor is much more supportive than a bed. Gravity pushes down, and the spine and head are completely supported.

The more you surrender, the heavier you feel physically, and the lighter the breath becomes. There is more space available inside because you have stopped trying to do anything. You are surrendering to the moment, to the floor, allowing yourself to be supported, trusting that you are safe as you rest here. Feel the pain gently dissipate.

AFFIRMATION: I TRUST MY BREATH TO MOVE ME AND TRIGGER THE HEALING RESPONSES IN MY BODY.

BREATH: ALTERNATE NOSTRIL BREATHING (NADI SHODHANA)

Let's re-visit this breath which was introduced in Chapter 6.

- Sit comfortably in a chair or on the floor with your hips spine supported.
- Make sure you sit up tall, feet flat on the ground. Let the shoulders drop down and back, opening the chest. Allow the eyes to be closed.
- Take your right hand and bend down then index and middle fingers.
- Place the right thumb against the right nostril and take a long, slow in-hale through the left nostril, filling belly, ribs and finally upper chest.
- Close off the left nostril with your ring finger as you lift the thumb and exhale fully through the right nostril.
- Then take another slow, deep inhale through the right nostril and repeat the pattern.
- This breath balances the sides of the body and the hemispheres of the brain; it calms the central nervous system.
- Take 10 long, slow inhales and 10 long, slow exhales.

MOVEMENTS/POSES: FROM THE LAST 10 DAYS

Put together the movements from the last 10 days and you have a short routine for yourself. Here's a list of them for your convenience and you can do them in any order, depending on how you feel and if you have pain. It's ideal to begin with a grounding meditative pose and to end with savasana or modified viparita karani.

1) Modified viparita karani
2) Pelvic tilting & savasana
3) Half-frog pose
4) Child pose
5) Cat/dog (variations, plus three-part breath)
6) One knee into chest (each side, plus)
7) Both knees into chest
8) Hamstring stretch with strap
9) Hip openers with strap
10) Half locust (each side)

CHAPTER 12: SIX MOVEMENTS OF THE SPINE

DAY 12

A supple body creates a supple mind and this makes sense since the spine is the center of the nervous system, where mind and body meet. Keeping the spine flexible and supple can keep you young and possibly lengthen your life span. Look at a yoga master such as B.K.S. Iyengar—at over 90 years of age, he is still lean, strong, and flexible.

Moving the spine keeps it from getting too rigid. If any part of the spine does become hardened or rigid, it affects the rest of the vertebrae as well as the extremities and impacts other bodily systems and functions.

The human spine is designed to move in six different directions: **forward and backward** (commonly called "flexion" and "extension"), **side to side** ("lateral") and **twisting** one way and the other ("rotation"). Each of these movements contribute to the overall health of the spine. They can gently realign the vertebrae by evening out the muscle tension, especially the lateral movements and the rotation. The greatest range of motion is usually found in the forward and backward flexion and extension.

The Cat and Dog stretches described in Chapter 5 are great for flexion and extension of the spine; Side Rolling and any gentle side stretches are great for lateral flexion and at the end of this chapter, you will find instructions for the Gentle Supine Spinal Twist. With modifications, these movements are accessible to any and all practitioners. The entire torso is expanded and contracted by breath and movement. This creates a wonderful internal massage for the abdominal organs, kidneys, liver, heart and lungs in particular. The lateral, side-to-side stretches are not necessarily a big movement, but they create a compression and release, massaging the ascending and descending colon and aiding in digestion. The side movements also stretch the intercostal muscles in between the ribs, and move any accumulated knots in the shoulder blades.

Twisting is important, but within this program we are going to use it conservatively. The spine is not really designed to twist very far from side to side. When we overdo our twisting, this creates undue tension on the ligaments in between the vertebrae, and they may become overstretched. The best way to work safely with twists is by elongating the spine on the inhale and then allowing the breath to ease you into the twist, rather than forcing your body into the position. This process can save your discs from wear and tear and any herniation.

Spinal rotation is akin to wringing out a wet washcloth; it helps us to gently squeeze the cerebral spinal fluid and move it around. The wringing motion also serves to squeeze out any toxins in the kidneys and abdominal organs. Twists are considered one of the best ways to balance and tonify the body and its systems.

You can always add in some of these movements of the spine during your workday: Sitting at your desk, use the arms or seat of your chair to support you in some flexion and extension (cat/dog) and/or gentle twisting (see 10-minute Desk Routine in the Appendices). When you stand waiting in a line, you can also practice small flexion/extension movements, tucking and releasing the tailbone with both feet planted on the ground at a hip-width distance.

If your spine is inflexibly stiff at 30, you are old; if it's completely flexible at 60, you are young...the only real guide to your true age lies not in years, or how old you THINK you feel, but...by the degree of natural and normal flexibility enjoyed by your spine throughout life.

-*Joseph Pilates*

AFFIRMATION: I MOVE SLOWLY AND MINDFULLY IN HEALTHY AND HEALING WAYS.

MOVEMENT: GENTLE SUPINE SPINAL TWIST

- On your back, let the knees be bent and the soles of the feet on the floor.
- Bring your arms out to the sides in a lazy T position.
- Take a deep inhale and feel your spine extend on the floor.
- As you exhale, gently let the knees fall over to the right as your head turns to the left. Inhale the knees and head back to center.
- Exhale and go in the other direction.
- Do this movement approximately 10 times with a soft gaze or eyes closed; focus inside using the breath.
- Stay aware of sensations that may come up and adjust accordingly.
- It doesn't matter how close to the floor the knees are or how far you can turn your head, just do what you can.

**I highly recommend this version for low-back safety while you are going through this program, even if you are capable of the more intense double-knee-down or knee-down versions.

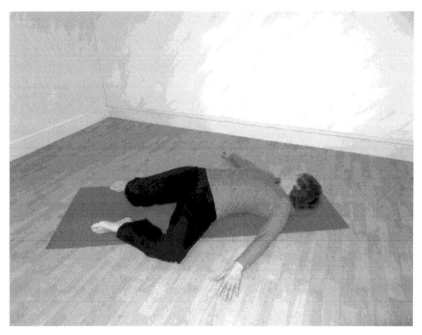

Gentle supine spinal twist

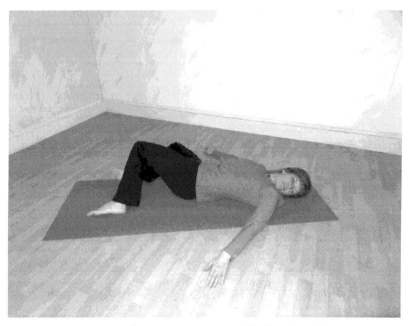

Let knees go over to one side, head to other.

CHAPTER 13: THE POWER OF GRAVITY

DAY 13

Gravity is the downward moving force that pushes against us every day as we stand or sit upright. It can be used to help us in many ways. Pushing our body up against gravity for a short period of time can strengthen muscles and even increase our bone mass. The **bridge pose** is fabulous for anyone with osteopenia or loss of bone density and may help to prevent these conditions; engage the abdominal muscles *first*, then lift the hips up and hold for a second or two before slowly releasing back down to the floor.

Anytime we lift an arm, a leg, or both at the same time, we create a natural resistance against gravity, thereby strengthening the body. Anytime we lie down on the floor or on our beds, we have an opportunity to literally "let go" and allow our muscles, tendons, and ligaments to rest. When your body is supported like this, there is no need for those muscles to be engaged at all; the bones can settle down and be heavy. Gravity offers us an incredibly healing experience if we surrender to it.

It takes no special skill or volume of muscle mass to allow gravity to work its magic on you. Your age, occupation, or socioeconomic background also don't matter. Gravity is a great equalizer—and it's working on all of us in every moment whether we like it or not, so why not use it to our advantage?

SURRENDER TO GRAVITY PRACTICE

- *Lie down on your back, on a mat or blanket on the floor and allow yourself to feel as if you are sinking into it.*
- *If your muscles, tendons, or ligaments are overstretched or super tight, it may actually take some practice to let go in your supine position.*
- *If the low back is sensitive, bend the knees and keep the soles of the feet on the floor or use a bolster under the knees.*
- *(Please note: do not try this on a bed – it will not offer the same support as a hard floor.)*
- *Place your hands on your belly and, with your eyes closed, allow the breath to flow easily in and out through the nostrils.*
- *As you inhale, allow the lungs to fill up as a balloon would, from the bottom to the top. Feel the belly push up into your hands, the sides of your ribcage expand and finally, feel the gentle lift in your upper chest.*
- *On the exhale, allow your lungs to empty out, again, as a balloon would deflate – emptying out from the top of your chest, feel the ribs contract in and finally, feel the belly sink back down and squeeze back towards the spine.*
- *And repeat with slow deliberate breaths.*
- *Let yourself feel the heaviness of your body and you relax more fully into the floor on each exhale.*

Notes:

- With the knees up and soles of the feet on the floor, you will still have to do some holding, so move toward stretching out your legs.
- You may find that if the back of the neck is very tight, a slight lift of the head will create a better position for the head and cervical spine, allowing the neck to lengthen and the chin to tuck in slightly towards the chest.
- You may also want to lie down on a rolled up blanket.

A complete release of the muscles, tendons, and ligaments creates space for the bones to move back into their normal and healthy alignment. Eventually, if you keep up this routine, you will become better and better at translating all of this to an upright position and when you stand, all of your work will pay off.

I would like to acknowledge Don Stapleton, senior Kripalu instructor and director of the Nosara Institute, for his informative and ground-breaking book, *Self-Awakening Yoga*. This work has truly changed my life and given me another approach for healing my own lower back and helping my private clients. You can link to the Nosara Institute website and book in here: www.nosarayoga.com and in the Print Resources section of this book. Don himself is proof of the healing power of gravity, having used a series of "movement inquiries" to heal himself from a serious case of scoliosis. Below is a gravity-friendly movement that is very healing for the spine.

AFFIRMATION: I OPEN TO NEW WAYS TO NURTURE AND HEAL MYSELF.

MOVEMENT: SIDE ROLLING

- Lie down on your right side with the right arm stretched out under the head and knees pulled up.

- Let your left hand rest on the floor, palm down in front of your chest for support.
- As you breathe out, gently allow the head to roll forward in front of the arm.
- If your forehead touches the floor, that's fine; if it doesn't, that's fine too.
- On your next inhale, gently lift the head and roll it up and over the arm.
- Let it be very heavy, as if you are moving through a very thick substance, like honey. Make it as effortless and lazy as possible.
- On your next exhale, let the head roll back behind the arm.
- The shoulder will want to open and probably the hip will slide back and open also. Go only as far as feels good for you.
- Inhale, do the lazy roll of the head up and over the arm again, and repeat.
- Try this 10 times on each side to help re-align the spine.

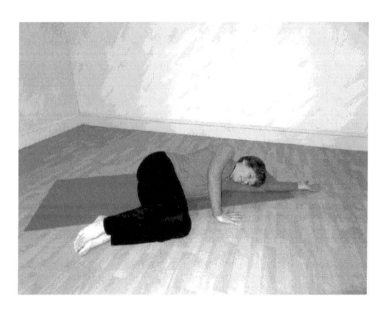

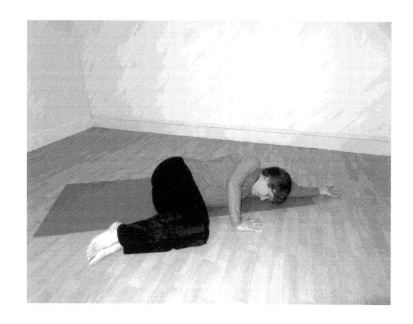

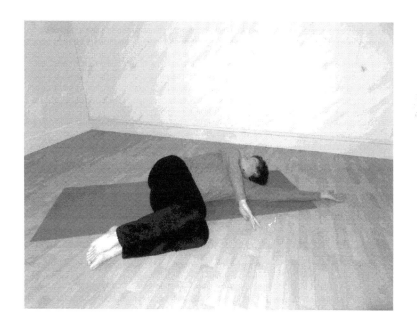

CHAPTER 14: CULTIVATE FLEXIBILITY

DAY 14

We may think of flexibility in terms of having a limber body, but I believe it's a state of mind as well. One kind of flexibility can enhance or create more in another area of your life. For instance, you must have been open to the *possibility* of stretching in order to buy this program. Somewhere in you, a voice said, "Yeah, I need to try something different, something more holistic. I'm going to go for it." And here you are -- stretching yourself mentally, creating space for new ideas. You are already more flexible than you think.

Stretching and strengthening are two opposite forces that are both necessary in order to cultivate more flexibility. Yoga is unique in that it both strengthens and stretches the body at the same time. Gentle stretching begins to break up the hard, knotted areas in the body that have become rigid. Depending on your age, habits, and previous health history (including genetics), you may find that certain areas of your body, particularly the spine, have frozen up and/or degenerated. They did not start out that way—we were all supple newborns at one time—and it is always possible to reclaim some of this flexibility.

Strength is a great thing to develop, but there are two sides to this coin. How many times have you seen the guys and gals in the gym who do nothing but strength training? Some of these people are very strong and have incredible arm muscles, ripples, six- and eight-packs, etc., but they are so tightly bound that everyday movement can be difficult or awkward. It doesn't have to be like that. You can look good and toned and be able to move with a normal amount of flexibility. There needs to be a balance.

The asana practice of yoga is unique in that almost every pose combines stretching and strengthening in different areas of the body at the same time. The breath can also contribute to your balance and flexibility. The inhale is an opportunity to expand and open the body; the exhale is an opportunity to release and let go of tension. The stretch happens on the exhale—it is an act of letting go.

AFFIRMATION: AS I OPEN MY BODY AND MIND, I BECOME MORE FLEXIBLE AND SUPPLE; MY LIFE FLOWS WITH EASE.

MOVEMENT: COBRA VINYASA

- Start in child pose, sitting back on the heels.
- On an inhale, lift up to all fours.
- On an exhale, bring the hips forward and down in front of you, bringing weight onto the hands, gently arching the lower back and opening the shoulders and chest.
- Hold a moment before you inhale back up to all fours.
- Exhale back down into Child pose.
- Move slowly and mindfully; keep eyes closed or a soft, unfocused gaze.
- Keep the movement going back and forth; follow the breath and hold when and where it feels appropriate.
- Focus on the connection between your breath and movement.
- Whatever fear or anxiety or stress you've been holding in your body, in your spine, let it all out with a sigh each time you exhale.

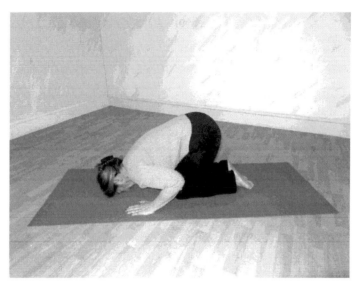

Cobra Vinyasa start

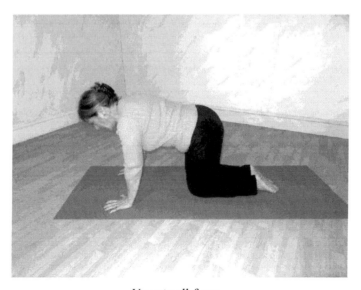

Up onto all-fours

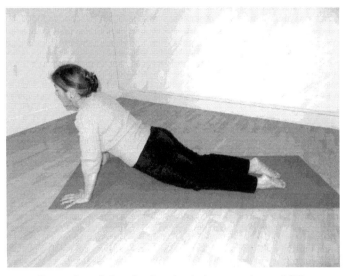

Down into Cobra (and go back down again to child)

MODIFICATION: SPHINX POSE INTO BABY COBRA

If you have wrist and/or knee issues, you can try this alternate pose:

- Lie on your belly and slide your arms back so that your upper body rises up and you end up on your elbows, gently arching the spine and reaching through the crown of the head.
- On the exhale, come back down to your belly.
- You can also try this: bring hands under the shoulders and push up into a "baby cobra" arch on an inhale
- Keep elbows in and slightly bent lower on the exhale.

CHAPTER 15: STRENGTHEN YOUR CORE

DAY 15

Your abdominal muscles wrap around your torso and connect to other muscle groups (back, thighs, hamstrings) which all work together to create a strong core and lower back.

Many women are more flexible than men in terms of range of motion, but women often have little or no core abdominal strength. This does not serve us. Flexibility without strength can lead to dislocation of joints, herniation of discs and other orthopedic injuries. The muscles, tendons, and ligaments work together to hold the bones in place. They need to be kept strong and flexible – not too tight, not too loose -- in order to do their job properly.

If your gluteus muscles around the low back and hips, the psoas and the quadrates lumborum are wound too tightly, they can be pulling your spine into misalignment and causing compression of the nerves. Clearly, we need to stay aware of this delicate balance between strengthening and stretching and find ways to accomplish this.

The first step is to test yourself to see what side of that equation is dominant in your body right now. And of course, some areas may be too tight, while others are too loose.

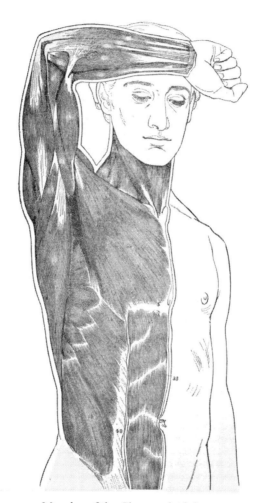

Muscles of the Chest and Abdomen

If you're too tight, you will probably answer yes to these questions:

Are you strong with significant muscle development?

Do you work out at the gym, but forget to stretch?

Do you get leg and foot cramps frequently (this can also be connected to lactic acid in the blood stream)?

<u>If you're too loose, these questions may pertain to you:</u>

Can you bend forward easily and touch your toes?

Are your hips open? Can you sit comfortably on a cushion or block in sukhasana (easy, cross-legged pose) with your knees reaching the floor?

Are you able to easily sit with legs straddled wide or do a complete monkey split down to the floor without any trouble?

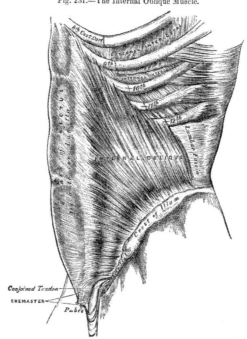

Fig. 231.—The Internal Oblique Muscle.

Side view of the oblique abdominal muscle

AFFIRMATION: AS I STRENGTHEN MY CORE ABDOMINAL MUSCLES, I STRENGTHEN MY LOW BACK.

MOVEMENT: BABY BRIDGES/BLOCK SQUEEZE

- Lie down on a yoga mat and let the soles of your feet come onto the floor, with the knees bent.
- Feet stay parallel and hip width apart with toes pointing straight ahead (to the extent you are able).
- Arms rest by your sides, palms down.
- Use a cushion or foam block and place it between your thighs for extra support/ resistance.
- Take a nice deep breath into the belly and as you exhale squeeze the block or cushion.
- **Feel your abs engage** as everything pulls in towards your belly button.
- Inhale and lift the hips up off the ground. Don't worry about how high you go up.
- Feel the knees stack over ankles. Exhale and slowly lower down. This will strengthen the abs and the low back. Try 10 of these.
- If this feels pretty good, try holding your hips up off the ground for another breath each time you raise them. No need to overdo this – keep the breath flowing and pay attention to sensation.

Bridge pose is contraindicated for Spinal Stenosis. Repeat Pelvic Tilting instead (Chapter 2).

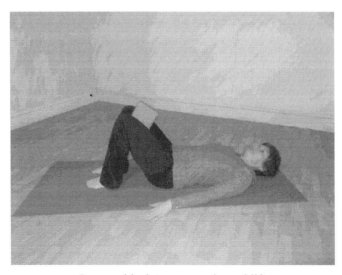

Squeeze block to engage abs and lift

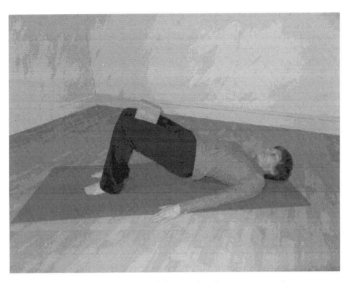

Baby bridge – keep ankles under knees as much as
possible as you slowly move up and down.

CHAPTER 16: THE ENERGETIC EXCHANGE

DAY 16

Whatever energy you put out into the universe is what you will get back. We've all experienced this in many different ways in our lives, but it goes even deeper than that. It's not just about the energy of "doing" – it's about the energy of "being." And sometimes it can feel difficult to just "be" if you have a lot of unresolved baggage you are carrying around from the past – usually childhood. Anger, fear, shame or guilt can be difficult to shake without a great deal of energetic guidance and support. This removal and purification of negative energy and obstacles is necessary in creating wholeness in your life.

It is much more than "reconditioning of the mind" – just deciding that you will think positive thoughts. That's a great idea, but if you have old energy under those words and thoughts that keeps you attached to your suffering, your injury, and/or accident and any anger, guilt, shame or blame that surround it, you will vibrate that out into the universe and that's what will be sent back to you. Your healing will never be complete and your pain will linger or keep coming back.

For most of us, the physical therapy aspect of recovery will not be difficult, but you must have the desire to heal, and be willing to do the work – to remember your own wholeness and keep going, even after this program. To do the removal and purification work, to train yourself or retrain yourself for success in healing your low back and break any possible addiction to your suffering and being a victim.

How can you do something like this? I would recommend finding a teacher and starting a daily meditation practice. Even the simple pranayams (breath exercises) I have included here in the book can be used for meditation. To take that a few steps further, you may want to study meditation more formally with a teacher. I feel most comfortable recommending my own teacher, Dr. Paul Muller-Ortega, but you will need to follow your heart on this one – just make sure that whomever you invest in working with has a great deal of first-hand experience and wisdom with which to guide you. Paul's contact information is listed in the resources section. If you are also interested in working with an amazing and inspirational teacher who can help you do the deeper work of transformation, again, I recommend my own teacher: Dr. Barbara DeAngelis – also listed in the Appendix.

> *All that we are is a result of what we have thought.*
> *—The Buddha*

This concept plays into chapter 8's discussion of lifestyle and habits. What are you exposing yourself to? What thoughts are you thinking? Are they negative? Are they positive? Are you in the present moment?

Make sure you keep these questions in mind each day, each hour and moment – make up index cards and carry them around it you have to. Instead of focusing on what you don't want, focus on what you really do want, open to gratitude – even for the pain. This may be a very challenging concept at first, but the pain was what got your attention and prompted you to take action. The pain is not "bad," it's just a message. It's a different way of approaching your healing, but try it and you may be surprised at the results.

This conditions the mind and preps the body for complete healing and requires faith—faith in yourself and in the fact that you are able to take control of your healing, that this is what the universe wants for you. My teacher says that it is impossible to feel grateful and to feel suffering in the same moment, within you. In other words, you can shift your "suffering" energy at any moment, by moving into gratitude, remembering all of the wonderful blessings you do have in your life.

AFFIRMATION: THE UNIVERSE IS CONSPIRING IN MY FAVOR. MY SPINE IS HEALED AND I AM FULL OF GRATITUDE.

MOVEMENT/POSE: BABY SUNBIRD ON EACH SIDE

- Start in child pose; take an inhale into the belly.
- Exhale, engage your abdominal muscles, lift up your right leg and reach back with your right toes, straighten the leg out and lift it.
- Don't worry about how high you lift, in fact, if you can keep your leg at hip level you will get stronger than if you lift it all the way up.
- Exhale and slowly release the leg back to the floor and come down to child pose again.
- Repeat 5-10 times with each leg.
- Focus on using the core abdominal muscles to control your movement up and down.
- Keep eyes closed or a soft gaze.

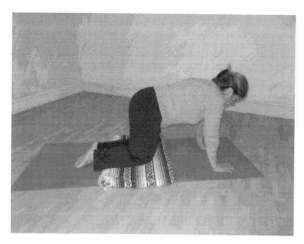

Baby Sunbird – start

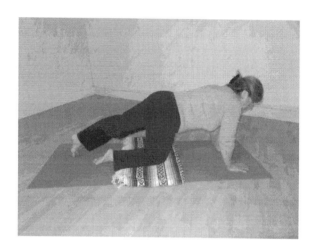

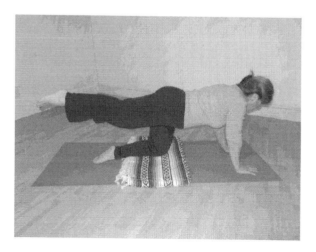

CHAPTER 17: CULTIVATE YOUR HEALING GARDEN

DAY 17

Think of your lower back as a garden that has perhaps been neglected over the years. Now that you have pain, you notice that your garden is overgrown with weeds; the soil is dry and devoid of nutrients. More oxygen, moisture, and fertilizer are necessary, along with a lot of faith and TLC. It's been 16 days since you began this program, how is your gardening project shaping up?

Hopefully you've gotten to the root of your problem and each day has been another exercise in weeding, fertilizing, sowing new and healthier seeds, caring for new sprouts. More knowledge about your body and a feeling of empowerment are natural byproducts; you are creating space for new growth that can be cultivated through new, healthier habits and eventually the benefits of a healthy body and life will be harvested.

Are you well nourished? Are you using all of your ingredients? Are you breathing deeply? Oxygen keeps the blood cells healthy, and promotes good circulation. Remember: as we take deep breaths in and out, the heart is massaged in between the lobes of the lungs.

Have you made any other changes in your lifestyle or nutrition? Have you noticed any other changes, not just physically, but emotionally, or mentally? In your interactions and relationships with others?

Lymph is another essential fluid in the body – part of the filtering or "weeding out" process if we keep thinking in terms of a garden.. Blood becomes tissue fluid which supplies nutrients to the cells; once this fluid absorbs the waste products of the cells, it is called lymph. Unlike the circulatory system, which has the heart to help it pump blood through the body, the lymphatic system has no pump. Its movement is dependent on the contraction and relaxation of muscle. External massage therapy or gentle bouncing of the body can help keep lymph from pooling and stagnating.

All the information you have been taking in each day can be considered new, healthy seeds that will replace the old myths and habits, whereas the movements you have been learning are something akin to fertilizer for your new, healing garden.

The day you began your 30-day journey, you really began to take care of yourself at another level. I want to acknowledge you for that—for being willing to try a new way, a new lifestyle, even just for 30 days. You know that what you were doing before this wasn't working, but change is never easy.

When you take a bold step forward in your life and begin with even one small change, others will follow. It probably won't happen in a neat or predictable fashion and will take a bit of getting used to. I can't tell you how you are feeling, but I can almost guarantee that some sort of transformation, however small, is taking place in your life right now.

Remember, nothing can grow or heal without attention to wholeness and completeness— and these things take time, so please be patient with yourself as you move forward with the program.

Let's use this chart to check in and see what you are noticing so far. Answer as honestly as possible to evaluate your own progress.

Progress Chart

ACTIVITY	NUMBER OF DAYS PRAC-TICED	LONG-TERM CHANGES NO-TICED (moods, reactions, interac-tions)	DESCRIBE HOW YOU FEEL IMMEDIATELY AFTER THIS PRAC-TICE
AFFIRMATIONS			
MOVEMENT/ STRETCHES			
BREATHING EX-ERCISES			
GUIDED VISUAL-IZATION CD (if you have it)			
JOURNALING			

AFFIRMATION: I CULTIVATE MY HEALING GARDEN DAILY WITH LOVING, POSITIVE THOUGHTS, DEEP BREATHS, AND MOVEMENT FROM MY CENTER.

MOVEMENT: GENTLE BOUNCES (LYMPHATIC WORKOUT)

- In standing, lift the heels a bit off the ground and gently bounce up and down, allowing your body to become very loose and heavy – or—keep feet on ground and gently bounce up and down.

- Let go of tension and let the gentle bounces relax you a bit more each time.
- It may also help to add a sound, like "ahhh"; open the mouth, let the jaw be loose and let out an "ahhh" as you bounce and jiggle.
- Do this for a minute or two.
- If your knees are healthy and you can take a bit more, do the same movement, only turn it into small jumps in which the whole foot comes slightly off the floor.
- This is not about how high you can jump, rather about shaking up the lymph and moving it around .
- Let yourself shake and make an "ahhh" sound along with the movement.

CHAPTER 18: DEVELOPING BODY AWARENESS

DAY 18

Our animal companions are very aware of their bodies. Cats walk lightly and surely, taking their time, enjoying sunshine and lots of naps. They curl up at will, roll around on their backs and rub up against anything that will scratch an itch, purring all the while. Dogs stretch themselves out, chew on some rawhide, play with toys, and jump up at any moment for a walk or a run, tail wagging, delighting in the attention that we pay them. Animals are completely connected and aware, completely in their bodies in each moment. Animals are wonderful teachers for us—they know how to feel good, go out of their way to do so, and don't judge themselves for it. Anything from a scratch to a hunger pang to a need for affection—they follow it with no apologies. They know how to be happy in their bodies, they know how to feel good. We can too.

Let's look at what you've done over the past 17 days:

1) You've brought your attention back into your body.

2) You've learned more about the anatomy of the spine and your injury.

3) You've started breathing more deeply and using the breath to heal your spine.

4) You've begun to condition and recondition the spinal muscles, and to cultivate your healing garden.

5) You've increased your awareness of gravity and how it can help in your healing process.

6) You've looked more closely at the root of the problem—how your injury came about and what habits you can change to prevent future injury.

7) You've brought awareness to your lifestyle, habits and the ways that overstimulation manifest in your life.

Breathe, Relax, Feel, Watch, and Allow

These are the five buzzwords (courtesy of Kripalu Yoga) that can remind you to focus inside: **breathe** deeply; **relax**, **feel** your body realign and shift, step back and **watch** the changes, and **allow** sensations to come up.

Deep breathing helps you to slow down. When we slow down, we relax. When we really begin to relax, our focus shifts from the head down into the physical body and we feel what is really going on inside. Sensation takes center stage for a change and our minds can have a rest as the parasympathetic nervous system takes over.

When we begin to feel ourselves fully in the present, using breath and relaxation, our witness consciousness begins to kick in. Witness consciousness is simply the ability to step back from yourself and "watch" what's going on— getting a new perspective on your body and your injury. It helps us to detach from identifying ourselves as the injury or pain itself so that we are able to simply experience it. In short, it gives us some leverage in the psychological realm. (I _feel_ pain versus I am _in_ pain.)

When we have this perspective, this new point of view, there is a sense of relief—things are not as bad as they seem. Knowledge is power. And if we take the time to know ourselves inside and out, we will be more open to allow our body's wisdom to guide us.

The best analogy I can offer is one that we are all quite familiar with— "not being able to see the forest for the trees." When we are stuck in a painful, uncomfortable state, our attention is quite narrow, intense, and focused. All we can see are a few trees—they seem very big, they surround us and perhaps make us feel trapped. If we take a few steps back, we can get some perspective on the situation. We take some control of our situation and our ego-mind and can step outside of those trees for longer and longer periods of time. Then and only then will we be able to see the whole forest—our whole bodies, our whole lives—and discover the root of our pain and injury which may be coming from something quite unexpected, such as a buried negative, emotional experience or trauma.

Through breath and body awareness, we begin to put the pieces of the puzzle together. We can see what it is that led up to this point and how we can better function in our daily lives in order to completely heal and prevent future pain and injury in the low back and other areas of the body.

Under conditions of heightened respiration, the heart, arteries, capillaries, veins, and lungs perform many days' labor in only a few hours. As blood circulation increases, basic nutrients are distributed to all the tissues in the body. Waste products accumulating in the cells are eliminated into the veins. Indeed, one can comprehend the significance of all forms of exercise by understanding this process alone. The body parts are moved merely to churn and stimulate the respiratory process.

-Swami Kripalu

AFFIRMATION: I BREATHE IN POSITIVE, HEALING ENERGY. I BREATHE OUT WHAT NO LONGER SERVES ME.

MOVEMENT: SUN BREATHS

- Widen your stance to more than hip-width while standing.
- Inhale, bring the arms up overhead and look up at your hands.
- Exhale, release the arms down and come into a squat with a large sigh or "Ha" breath.
- Let your downward motion be heavy and sloppy. Let go of control and of "trying."
- Enjoy the release as if you are "throwing down" all of those burdens you carry around on your shoulders.
- Allow the inhale to lift you and propel your arms up overhead and the exhale to release the shoulders, neck, and upper body.
- Repeat this at your own pace, 5 to 10 times.
- If your back is currently sore or bothering you, come down into the squat with a straight spine—don't bend forward.

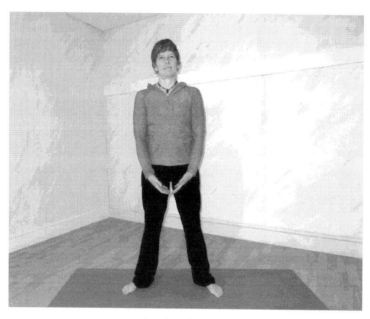

Sun breath start;

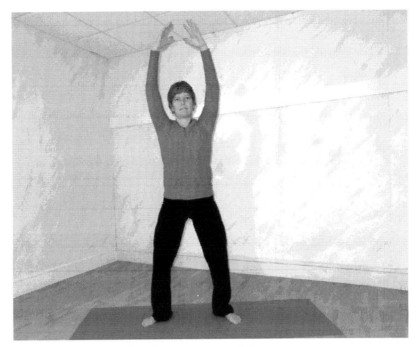

Sweep arms up on inhale.

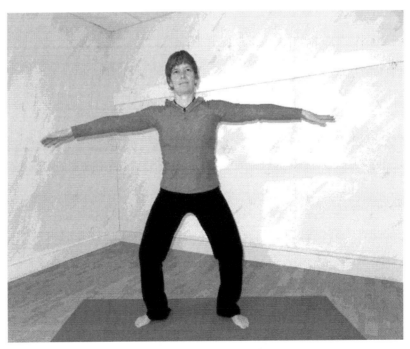

Exhale and let arms drop down.

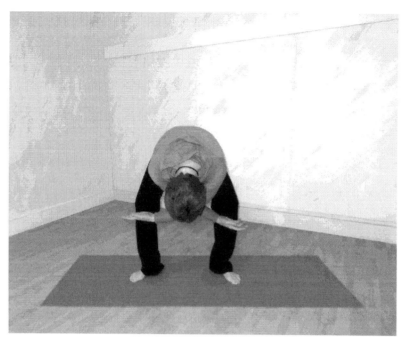

Fold forward, come back up and repeat.**

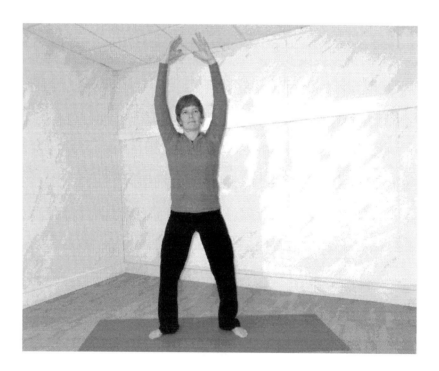

** If this is too much on your lower back, just let the arms release down and squat, don't fold forward.

CHAPTER 19: GETTING LEVERAGE

DAY 19

We already talked about the force of gravity and how we can use it in our favor. We also need to maintain good posture -- keeping our vertebrae stacked in proper alignment in order to fully support the weight of the upper body and balance the torso over the hips and legs when walking or sitting. Our task is even more difficult in our modern world of stress, overwork, and bad posture and body position at our computers, desks, and in the car. The odds are already against us in terms of keeping a healthy curvature in the spine. We need *leverage* to help us. While witness consciousness gives us leverage in the psychological realm, body mechanics gives us this leverage in the physical realm.

Using your body weight for everyday safety

Did you know that the Lumbar 4 and 5 vertebrae carry the majority of the weight of the upper body, and that half your body weight is above the waist?

It's no wonder that this area (along with the Sacroiliac or "SI" joint) is so prone to injury.

When you bend over at a 90-degree angle from the hip, the spinal muscles must work extra hard to hold you there. On top of this, anything you lift or carry increases the required tension to hold your body in a forward bend. This is also one of the main reasons that my program steers away from forward bending. I don't recommend forward bends if you have any kind of low-back weakness or injury—and most especially if you have osteoporosis and/or osteopenia. The majority of vertebral fractures occur in forward bending motion. Activities like shoveling snow and vacuuming can be devastating to the lower back if you forget to bend your knees.

Of course there are plenty of everyday activities you do in which you need to bend forward. Here are some tricks you can use to leverage yourself. These are simple adjustments you can make, inside and out, that lessen the weight needed to keep your upper body in a safe position:

Bend your knees before you reach down to lift an object. This immediately takes the stress off the low back, tipping the sacrum forward instead of back. If we move too fast, we may forget. Take a breath before you reach forward, twist, and/or lift a child, animal, or object.

Lift with the legs -- utilizing legs and large muscles will diminish the stress on the back.

Use a step stool. Have a small stool handy around the house to get yourself up to the proper level to reach for and lift items. You may also use it to put one foot up as you perform certain activities. This asymmetrical position can take the pressure off the low back. A real life example: Put one foot up on the curb when you pump your own gas.

Use a hand on a flat surface to support you as you lean forward. Real life examples: wiping the table, brushing your teeth.

Stand close to the object you're lifting and face it squarely. Don't reach out and forward or twist the spine *even slightly* while attempting to lift

118

something. The ligaments that hold the vertebrae in place are not meant to move very much or very far.

Minimize twisting – Pivot your feet or move your entire body to decrease stress on your back.

Push an object – Pushing an object (vs. pulling) increases your leverage against the weight of the object and thus is easier on your back.

Tighten your abdominal muscles – reduce strain to the back before you lift or move an object, by tucking your tailbone which engages your abdominal muscles.

Beware of vacuuming and shoveling activities – these are very tough on the low back!! Bend those knees and get yourself proper equipment to use – yes, there are "ergonomic" shovels. Maybe it's time for a snow blower if you live in Midwest or Northeastern U.S.

Incorporate some of these ideas into your daily routine and see if you notice a difference. See what other new and creative ways/props you can come up with to support yourself. Ergonomics also plays a key role in maintaining good body mechanics.

AFFIRMATION: I SEE MY WHOLE SELF, COMPLETELY HEALED.

POSE: CHAIR DOG (USING A WALL OR THE BACK OF A CHAIR) OR DOWNWARD FACING DOG

- Stand with hands on the wall or chair and slowly walk back until your body is in a 90-degree "L" position or a wider angle.
- Your back should be relatively flat, pelvis and sacrum tipping forward, tailbone up. If your lower back is rounding, you have bent over too far.
- Notice your hamstrings. If they are really tight, you can bend the knees to alleviate any extra pressure on the low back.
- You can also "walk your dog" by pedaling the feet heel to toe, back and forth; this gives the calves a good stretch.

- If you're in pretty good shape and are familiar with regular Downward Facing Dog, go ahead and come into the pose on a sticky mat away from the wall or chair.

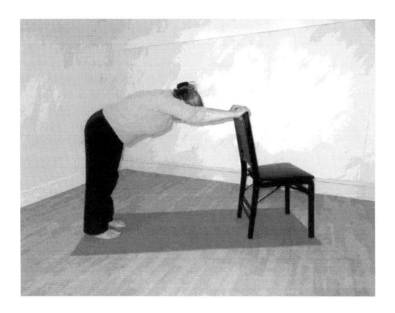

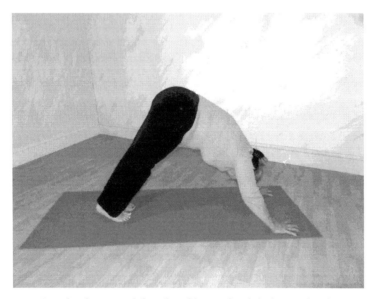

Regular downward dog (bend knees for tight hamstrings);
<u>A little trick:</u> If your hands slip on the mat, use a yoga strap under them.

CHAPTER 20: BODY MECHANICS TO STAND & WALK

DAY 20

Today you have another opportunity to observe yourself and your habits and cultivate good posture. You will need a long mirror to look at yourself from the front and side. Without trying to do anything different, stand in your natural stance in front of the mirror.

- *From the front, how far apart are your feet ?*
- *Do you notice any bowing of the leg bones?*
- *Are your hips even or does one look higher than the other?*
- *Are you standing with weight evenly distributed across the foot?*
- *Do your toes point straight ahead, or do they fan out to the sides? Or do you have "pigeon toes" angling in? Are your knees knocking together?*

Standing with toes turned out is usually a sign that your hips naturally rotate out; your inner thighs are probably not very strong but you have good flexibility, and your ilio-tibial band on the outer upper leg is probably very tight and overcompensating for the inner thigh weakness. Long-term, this is not good for the knee joint -- you may find yourself with torn cartilage in the medial (inside) meniscus. This is just one typical of how everything is interrelated.

- *Do you lean in on the insides of your feet or out on the outsides?*

This will be much more noticeable was you have someone watch you walk, but take a look at the bottom of your shoes and notice where the heels are most worn down – inner or outer? We all tend to either pronate or supinate unless we have special orthotics in our shoes to help us. Consider seeing a specialist to have custom orthotics made; these will most likely help to alleviate hip and low-back pain.

You may need a friend or family member to help you evaluate your stance from the side.

- *From the side, do your ear, shoulder, hip, and ankle should make a relatively straight line? If they don't, notice what's out of place.*
- *Try tucking your tailbone underneath you and feel and see what happens to your hips and spine.*
- *Keep the knees soft (not locked) and legs strong, arms are relaxed at the sides.*

Here are some simple adjustments you can make to help your body mechanics and posture:

- ***Spread your feet to at least hip width*** *to give yourself a sturdy base to lift from.*
- ***Keep torso centered over hips*** *to encourage the natural stacking of the vertebrae in a healthy "S" curve. The spine is very strong in its natural alignment and you will be able to lift anything safely with knees bent.*

When the tailbone tucks and the pelvis moves into a neutral position under the torso, this engages the **abdominal muscles**, and the **gluteal muscles.** You will also feel the kneecaps lift as the **quadriceps** engage. It's much easier to open the chest and lift through the sternum once you have tucked and engaged those abdominal muscles. I also find it much easier to stand comfortably when I move into this alignment.

Here's another version of the above "tailbone tuck" movement to help us feel our abdominal muscles and realign our standing posture.

AFFIRMATION: I HONOR MYSELF AND MY BODY DAILY IN EVERY CHOICE, EVERY BREATH, EVERY MOVEMENT.

POSE: MOUNTAIN WITH FOAM BLOCK

- In standing, use a block or sturdy cushion.
- Place it between your thighs.
- The block will help you to find your "hip width distance" for the feet.
- Squeeze the block and feel the tailbone tuck, abs engage, pelvis moves into a neutral position, and the hips are right under the torso.
- Notice how much easier it is now to lift the sternum and let the shoulders come back and down. This opens the chest and helps to reduce any kyphosis in the upper back that may be developing from hunching over a computer, steering wheel, etc.

- Now on an inhale, lift your arms up and out to the sides and overhead.
- Drop your shoulders away from the ears. Find the position for your arms that is most comfortable and try holding them there for a minute.
- Take another breath into the belly and notice your core abdominal muscles.
- Notice if you are lightly squeezing that block or cushion or if you released little bit.
- Notice also how your spine moves back into alignment when the tailbone tucks under.

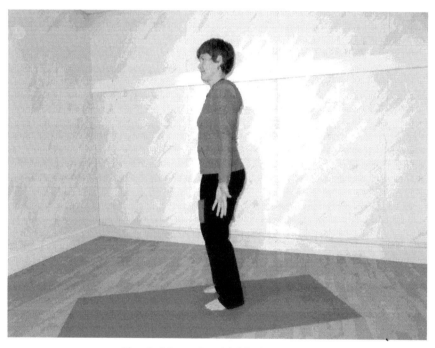

Simple Mountain with block squeeze

Obviously, during the day as you are out and about, at work, running errands, picking up your kids, etc., you won't be able to carry a block around between your thighs to help you, but you can keep awareness about your posture. Notice how you stand in line at the grocery store or at the bank. How about when you hold your child in your arms—which hip do you favor? How do you carry bags of groceries? Are you able to notice how you overcompensate? Do you shift the hips side to side, back and forward?

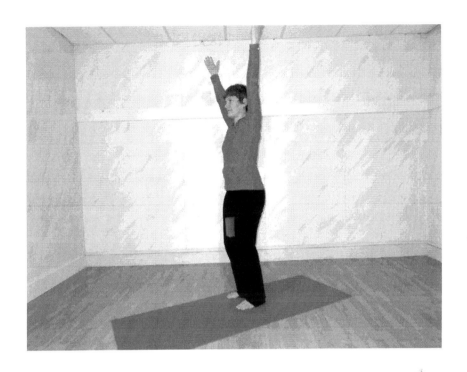

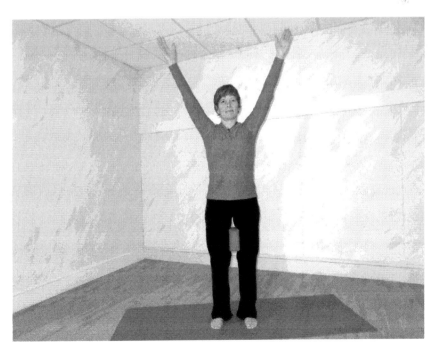

All these habits can have a cumulative effect over time. It's a fact that if your hips are out of alignment, one of your legs is probably a bit shorter than the other (this is usually a muscular issue which can turn into an orthopedic issue over time. Misaligned hips and uneven legs will lead to spinal problems, especially lower back pain. If you favor one side, try using the other.

Doing a walk evaluation can be a bit more tricky – it would be great to have a friend watch you, ask these questions, and make notes for you:

- *When you walk, do you lead with your head?*
- *Do you stand up straight or do you hunch forward as you move?*
- *How do you hold and move your arms?*
- *Do you walk with toes pointed straight ahead or do toes turn in or out?*
- *Do you put one foot straight out in front of you, rolling heel to toe and then placing the other foot out in the same way? If not, then how would you describe your foot position?*
- *Do you stride easily moving legs back and forth?*
- *Do you bounce up and down and you walk?*
- *Do you keep a bend in your knees as you make strides or are your legs more rigid?*
- *How would you describe your hip movement as you walk?*

You can apply most of the same principles of stacking joints in walking as in standing. Ideally, you want the joints to come through a stacked position at certain points in your gait. If you focus on keeping the toes pointed straight ahead and walking heel to toe, this will help to keep the ankles strong – the ripple effect works its way up into the knee and finally up into the hip joint. You want the knee to track back and forth over the foot and ankle, with no twisting.

Let's look at what happens when you walk with your feet turned out – go ahead and just sit this way for a moment – what happens to the knees? They turn out also-- the stacking over the ankles disappears, as does the stability for this joint. If your feet are turned out and your knees torque out to the sides as you walk, there will be imbalance and weakness in these two areas and the hips will end up having to over-compensate somehow. You may find yourself shifting more weight onto one side, making yourself lopsided and forcing the hip to rotate in an unhealthy way. This can wear down the joint cartilage.

By continuing to walk the way you are, you are throwing off your hips and therefore your spinal alignment. A positional therapist, orthopedist, or orthotic specialist will also be able to tell you whether one of your legs is shorter than the other, usually by watching you walk barefoot or by measuring the length of your legs while you are lying on an exam table.

Custom orthotics are created directly from a foam impression made of your foot, and are usually covered or reimbursed by health insurance. Generic orthotics are also available in medical supply stores and online for much less. Look for Aertrex by Lycos. Dr. Scholl's also makes low-end orthotics -- not nearly as effective as the medical generics or the customized orthotics. (See the Resources section for more information.) **Ladies – one more time – please get off of those high heels! Your spine, hips and feet will thank you.**

Even if your standing habits are not the direct cause of your current discomfort, looking at those habits and adjusting accordingly can only help in the healing process, to keep you in good alignment for the future, preventing other injuries.

Since we all are tighter on our dominant side, it may feel as if one leg is a little bit shorter than the other. This is usually a muscular situation as opposed to a bone abnormality. With some traction and hip balancing, this situation can usually be alleviated. See the Resources section for more information on Positional Release Therapy.

CHAPTER 21: THE ERGONOMICS OF SITTING

DAY 21

While "body mechanics" refers to how we move and arrange our bodies in the performance of everyday tasks, "ergonomics" is about our movement and position in relation to the objects and items we use. Now that you have begun to stretch and strengthen your back, let's make sure that all you've done for yourself is not undone by bad habits.

Good spinal alignment and joint alignment begins with "**stacking**"—that is, feeling your joints line up, feeling your vertebrae sitting one of top of another with your head resting comfortably on top of the spinal column.

Our straight-backed chairs are generally not designed to put us into a good spinal alignment, but perhaps you have the good fortune to work for a company that is concerned about the ergonomic set-up of its employees. If so, you may have an office chair, ergonomic mouse, and other props and paraphernalia that make it easier and more comfortable to sit at your desk and in front of your computer. You're way ahead of the game.

Let's take a regular chair and look at what you can do to turn it into an excellent support for your spine, without any fancy cushions or props:

Sit in the chair with feet flat on the ground and notice how it positions your spine. Actually, make sure your feet are able to be flat as you sit. Try sliding forward and sitting on the edge of your chair. If this still doesn't work for your feet, try another chair (preferably an office chair with a pneumatic lever which allows you to adjust the height).

Does the back of the chair meet your spine in a comfortable place or do you have to lean back farther than 90 degrees to have any support? Can you sit with shoulders back and chest open? Notice the position of your lower back—ideally the tailbone is tipped up and back. We want to avoid rounding the lower back.

Is your head hanging forward in front of your torso? If so, this is putting undue stress on the upper back and neck muscles and will in turn affect the mid- and low back as the spine struggles to hold the weight of the head. (The average human head weighs about 12 pounds— that's heavy!)

- To adapt regular straight-back chairs, get a cheap, standard bed pillow from the dollar store. Roll up the bottom of one end and place it in the curve of your low back. Sit back and notice how the roll supports your low back while the rest of the flat pillow supports you as you sit upright in a chair. This is a very easy and economical solution for improving your posture in a non-ergonomic chair. (Thanks to Lee Albert, NMT, for this tip.)

- For office chairs, if your office does not have decent desk chairs, use either a bed pillow or any kind of small, bean bag cushion, inflatable cushion; or a regular lumbar cushion. Place it in the small of the back.

- If you sit at a lab station or workbench and must use a stool, make sure it has a back to it. You may be able to use the rolled-up pillow behind you for some support here.

- <u>Try also using a wedge cushion</u> which elevates the hips slightly at an angle and tips you forward a bit. No matter what your age, if you have to sit in a lot of non-ergonomic chairs, a wedge cushion is always a good investment. **Relax-o-Back** makes a very sturdy foam cushion with a washable cover. The company has been around for years; I have one of their cushions and it's a lifesaver. Their wedges also have a little cutout area for the tailbone. You can also use this for support on a couch if the cushions are sturdy enough.

- Some fancier ergonomic office chairs will adjust to pitch you forward at a slight angle and you may not need the wedge.

Your work space

Whether sitting at home at the kitchen counter, at your desk at work, or at your workbench, your chair is just the first part of good ergonomics. We also need to look at where your arms, hands, and feet are positioned.

Arms are ideally bent at a 90-degree angle, with elbows tucked in close to the ribs, so that the shoulders can relax down from the ears. If the angle is less than 90, you need to raise the height of your chair or put some sort of comfortable lift or cushion on the seat. If it's more than 90 degrees, try to raise the height of the table or desk or lower your chair. This is especially important if you do a lot of typing at your computer.

Hands should be able to rest on a keyboard or surface with ease, facing straight ahead with no reaching.

Feet should always be flat on the floor, unless you are using a wedge cushion or your chair tilts you forward. In this case, it might be necessary to purchase an angled foot rest. *Do not cross your legs!* This is bad for the hips and low back and constricts circulation in the legs.

When you hold your extremities at a comfortable angle while seated (no reaching, no scrunching up of shoulders), you are taking pressure off the spine; the head is no longer inclined to pull you forward and the neck is protected.

Ergonomic items

If you need a good office chair at home, try one of the big office warehouses like Staples or Office Max. These places are great because you can "try before you buy." Besides the ergonomic chairs, there are also ergonomic **computer keyboards** shaped to a more natural position for the hands (turned in a bit). Microsoft makes one of these keyboards, but there are other brands out there that are just as good and more reasonably priced.

An ergonomically correct **computer mouse** can be a lifesaver if you are married to a computer most of the day. My favorite is by Logitech; it has a red tracking ball to move the cursor around and two clickers on either side, and my hand rests comfortably on the shaped surface. Consider a **gel wrist rest** for when you use your mouse, and if you have to read documents as you type, use a **document holder**. Also, take a look at your work phone situation—do you have a **headset** available for long conversations? How far do you have to reach to pick up your phone and dial if you have a land line? You may simply need to reposition your phone to avoid a long reach.

If your computer monitor is too low for your eye level, set it up on one or two phones book or something comparable and sturdy.

In the car and on a plane

Your seat height and position have similar guidelines whether sitting in a chair at a desk or at the dinner table, or doing any other activities that involve sitting in a chair:

Seat Position (forward/back)-- Arms are ideally bent at a 90-degree angle, with elbows to the sides and hands gently holding the wheel at either 10am and 2pm or 4pm and 8pm, so that the shoulders can relax down from the ears. If the angle is less than 90, you are too close in to the wheel and need to push your seat back. If it's more than 90 degrees, slide your seat forward to be closer to the wheel.

Legs should be extended comfortably in front of you with a slight bend in the knee. You shouldn't have to reach too far with your foot to press the pedals, in fact, the heel needs to rest on the floor of the car so that you can easily switch from gas to brake.

Seat Height -- You will also need to adjust the seat height to help with your hold on the wheel – I have usually found that most seats are adjusted too low. The height of the wheel should not be above your shoulders. If you are short in stature, you may need an extra seat cushion under you to lift you up an extra inch or two.

Seat Back Reclining Angle – This has got to be the most misused "comfort device" ever. So many clients I see recline their seat back too far, especially in sportier cars. This throws everything off – it forces your arms to straighten and reach further forward as your spine rounds into the lower part of the seat; your shoulders are hunched completely, and the head also reaches out in front of the shoulders and the spine, especially when hands are placed on top of the wheel.

I would try to keep your seat back as close to upright as possible or work yourself back up there by degrees if it initially feels uncomfortable – in the long run this could really alleviate neck, shoulder and low-back discomfort when driving.

On a plane, you can also do some things, bring some props to help you have a more comfortable seated position and reclining position. Though you generally cannot control the height of the seat, you can bring a wedge cushion along with you to sit on. Likewise, you can bring a lumbar support cushion for behind the back or sometimes one of those small "koosh" (bean bag) pillows is even better because it will shift and mold to your lumbar spinal curve for better support. You can also bring a thin bed pillow along and use it as described a couple of pages ago – folded on one end and placed in the small of the back with the rest of the pillow supporting your spine and neck .

Another idea is to use the small airplane pillow in the small of your back instead of under your head – or ask for two, so that you can support both areas. I personally find that it's my neck that needs more support than my head and I have one of those Bucky™ buckwheat neck cushions that I carry on board. You will need to experiment with what works best for you.

What is O.S.H.A. and how can it help me?

The Occupational Safety and Health Administration (**OSHA**) is a government organization within the U.S. Department of Labor. OSHA establishes standards for ergonomic safety, including those at computer workstations that must be met by your employer. If you are in need of any of the aforementioned ergonomic items at work, discuss this with your supervisor and/or human resources representative.

http://www.osha.gov/SLTC/etools/computerworkstations/

If it's possible, get a professional to do an ergonomic evaluation of your work station. Many times, larger corporations will hire a contractor to come in and do this for all employees. Sometimes it's very hard to notice how you are sitting or leaning and whether or not there are problems. As part of my crusade for healthy ergonomics, I offer this service myself, traveling to clients' workplaces. I do in-depth evaluations of each employee and their workstation and equipment and make recommendations on what each needs to do or buy in order to be ergonomically correct and safe. Please contact me directly if you or your company is interested in this service.

AFFIRMATION: I MOVE INTO GREATER AWARENESS AROUND MY EVERYDAY HABITS.

MOVEMENT: VICTORY SQUATS

- Stand with feet wider than hips, toes turned out slightly.
- Inhale arms up overhead, dropping the shoulders away from the ears.
- On an exhale, sink down into a wide squat, coming down with a straight spine.
- Imagine there is a 10-pound weight attached to your tailbone and keep it tucked slightly.
- Bring the arms down at right angles, palms facing in towards the head.
- Inhale, straighten the legs, and reach up to the sky.
- Repeat 5 to 10 times, increasing as it feels right to you.

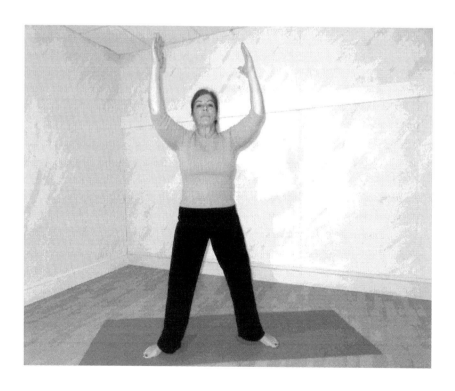

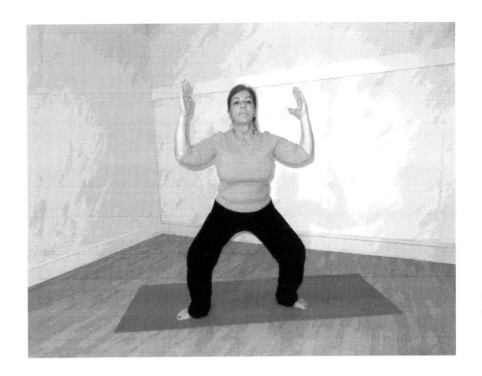

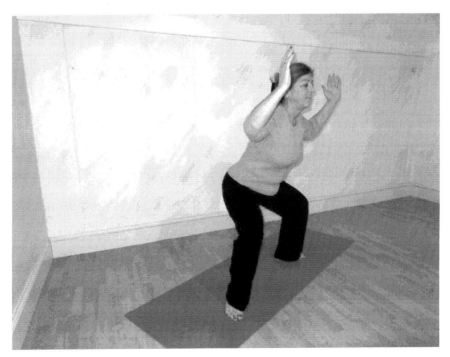

Don't stick out your tailbone and lean forward like this! Stack those joints.

CHAPTER 22: THE ERGONOMICS OF SLEEP

DAY 22

We all spend one-third of our lives asleep, and it always amazes me when I find out how many people are unaware or simply ignoring that they are still sleeping on a 20-year-old mattress with a permanent dip carved out of the middle area. This kind of a bed is the perfect place for spinal problems to develop or worsen!

Ergonomics, as we discussed in the last chapter, has to do with designing and arranging things people use for optimum interaction benefits. I don't think I've ever seen "sleep" linked with "ergonomics" before, but I am connecting them here because I believe it is a very important area that is often over-looked when it comes to spinal pain and recovery.

The science and design of mattresses and other sleep props has come a long way in the past twenty years. There are now many styles of mattresses and materials to choose from including natural foam, latex foam, memory foam and air chambers, and that's a good thing because we are all unique in our needs and comfort levels. Perhaps allergies are an issue; perhaps you go for the soft pillow-top, or maybe you need a very firm mattress. There is something out there for everyone.

Whatever your preferences, take a long, hard look at your current mattress. Take off all the sheets and really look. Try it out as if you're in a show-room. Does it still have enough firmness and support? Is it sagging in the middle? If you have one of those air mattresses (Sleep by Numbers), have you tried different settings? Have you flipped or turned your mattress within the last few years? If you haven't, that might be a first step. Take a trip to your local mattress store and try out some of the new ones just for the heck of it. A new mattress could be a great investment in your healing process.

And what about your pillow? How old is it? Is it made of foam, feather or microfiber material? Does it support your neck well enough? Test it out, lying on your side and then again lying on your back, two very different scenarios. Could you use a new one? Go ahead and buy it – again, in the bigger picture investing in a new pillow for under $100 and probably much less, is a small price to pay on the path to a healthier, pain-free spine.

If you have lower back pain, do you use anything to elevate your knees in bed when you sleep—perhaps a foam wedge, a bolster, or another pillow? This will take pressure off the low-back area and hips. One of those long and bulky body pillows helps many people to sleep more comfortably on their side. When you hug it between knees and elbows, it keeps the knees at about hip width and elbows apart, also easing shoulder and neck tension.

AFFIRMATION: I SURRENDER TO THE GIFT OF SLEEP AND RE-CEIVE ITS BENEFITS.

MOVEMENT: SACRAL MASSAGE

- Lie down on your back, bring knees into the chest and gently wrap your arms around them, hands below the knees or folded under them.
- Slowly begin to make a circle with the knees and bring them around, using your breath and hands to guide them.
- You will feel a gentle massaging of your sacrum as it pushes against the floor
- Make circles for at least 5 breaths in one direction and then pause and switch to 5 breaths in the other direction.

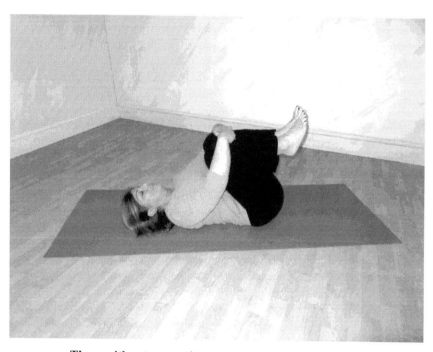

Those with osteoporosis or osteopenia should proceed gently and with caution.

CHAPTER 23: REST IS GOOD MEDICINE

DAY 23

Today is about resting. By that I mean "holistic" resting—not just getting a good night's sleep, but finding ways to cultivate a balance between rest and activity during the daytime hours. Even as you work, notice how you might make things easier and healthier for yourself, alternating between different activities. Give yourself a cut-off time for each activity. Sit at the computer for an hour and then make sure you get up and take a walk. Stretch whenever you can. Change your position frequently. Take some deep breaths. Do cat and dog stretches in standing or sitting in your chair. Put some music on and move to it for 5 minutes.

There are also nourishing practices you can try that may enhance your rest when you do take it, or help to keep you energized but calm. Certain foods and beverages soothe and others stimulate; we all know this intuitively, but we may not think about it.

Practice the art of napping. Take a 20 minute cat-nap in the middle of the afternoon. Many of us have a natural inclination for a short "siesta" – this is not wrong or bad or lazy. And in fact, there is one wonderful Ayurvedic practice that involves lying down on your left side right after you eat for at least 10 minutes. This places the stomach and intestines in a position that promotes peristalsis -- the digestion and movement of food through your system. It can prevent bloating and indigestion. Try it and see what happens.

Take rest; a field that has rested yields a bountiful crop.
—Ovid

Sleeping soundly

While a little rest during the day can be very healing and rejuvenating, getting a good night's sleep is essential. If you have trouble sleeping, the different breathing techniques we've gone over (in particular, three-part breath and alternate nostril breathing) can help you calm the mind and body before you sleep. Sometimes a few gentle Cat and Dog stretches before bed will help—or side rolling on the floor; perhaps a cup of warm milk with a sprinkle of cinnamon will do the trick. The Ayurvedic herb called "ashwaganda" is also associated with sound sleep and rejuvenating the adrenal glands.

In the sleep state, our brain produces several different kinds of brain waves; this is actually how the electrical activity in the brain is measured. The wave frequencies are listed in Hertz or cycles per second.

In our waking state, our brain waves are cycling at 14-30Hz; these are Beta waves. When we are relaxed, daydreaming, or engaging in creative activities, Alpha waves are prevalent; they cycle a bit slower, at 8-13Hz. In our dreaming state, as well as when we meditate and our subconscious mind is engaged, the cycles slow even more, to 4-7Hz; these are Theta waves. Finally, in a deep sleep state, we are unconscious and not dreaming; Delta waves are active at 0.5-6Hz.

In order to completely rest the body, mind, and spirit and promote deep healing, we need to reach the Theta and Delta brain-wave levels and allow ourselves to stay there for hours, without disturbance. Of course, the ideal amount of sleep needed varies from person to person, but the general rule of thumb is 8 hours. The brain can and does function in one or more frequency at a time; they generally overlap.

The best cure for insomnia is to get enough sleep.
—W.C. Fields

Here's an example of how we are directly connected to nature and dependent on her for our healing processes, and where sleep fits in: When we're outside in the sun, we absorb vitamin D into our systems; vitamin D helps us absorb calcium; calcium stimulates the pineal gland, located just behind the middle of the forehead (the location of the "third eye" or the "sixth chakra"); and the pineal gland is responsible for triggering the production and release of melatonin into the system. The production of melatonin in turn stimulates the production of cortisol (to control stress and store fat) and adrenaline (which controls stress and regulates blood sugar).

So if we don't get enough vitamin D or calcium, melatonin is not produced in the necessary quantities. That will create an inability to fall asleep easily. We are very sensitive beings—if one piece of the puzzle is missing, everything gets thrown out of whack. It's a domino effect.

Pain is another big block to our rest. If your low back pain is keeping you awake, you may end up with other medical issues from sleep deprivation. This is a tricky situation if you want to avoid prescription, narcotic pain killers. I recommend avoiding them whenever possible, but sometimes, they are a must if you are in an extreme situation and have not been getting enough sleep.

Bottom-line: Rest is one of the main ingredients for any physical healing, and especially for the spine. If you don't get rest, you will have a very hard time breaking your cycle, restoring, rejuvenating and letting some deep healing take root.

AFFIRMATION: MY SLEEP IS DEEP AND SOUND; I WELCOME THE REST I NEED TO HEAL AND WAKE UP REFRESHED AND RENEWED.

MOVEMENT: COMPLETE ROLLING SIDE TO SIDE

- On your back, bring the knees into the chest, just as in the sacral massage, and place your hands on your kneecaps as if you were holding onto them like knobs.
- Gently allow your body to roll all the way over to one side and then roll back through center and over to the other side.
- Let the body be very heavy and the movements slow and sloppy.
- Feel any tension releasing into the floor.
- Eyes are closed or unfocused in a soft gaze.

**(Those with osteoporosis or osteopenia should proceed gently and with caution.)

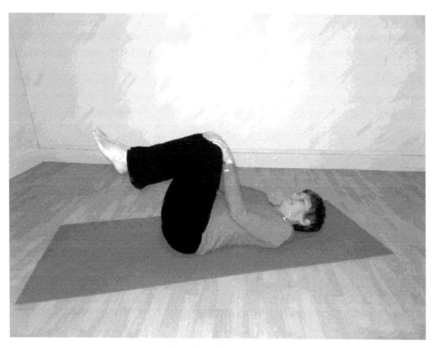

Hands on kneecaps

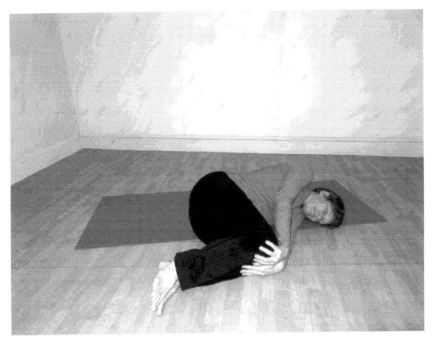

Roll all the way over to one side.

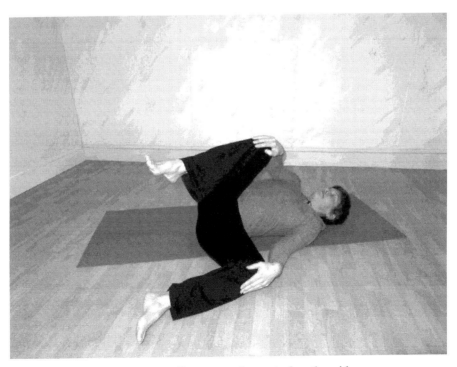

Let the knee pull you up and over to the other side;

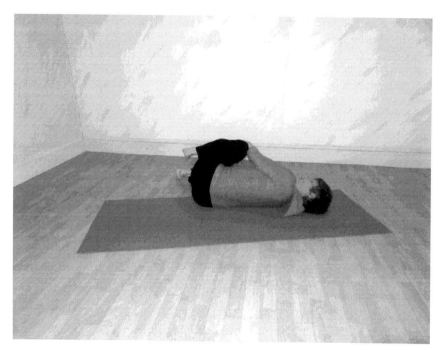

And begin again.

CHAPTER 24: THE WISDOM OF THE BODY

DAY 24

Our bodies are amazing feeling, breathing, and thinking machines. We don't need to be awake to be alive—our lungs know when we need to breathe, our bodies tell us what they need and when. Hungry, thirsty, tired -- as long as we are paying attention, our bodies are constantly sending us messages to keep us in good health. All we have to do is listen.

Unfortunately, many times our brain gets in the way of our body's wisdom; we have a lot of mental chatter and activity to contend with. Because we live in a world that seems to be moving faster and faster each day, imposing more deadlines, throwing more and more external sensory stimulation our way, this takes our attention away from the sensations going on in our bodies. The chatter rarely contains good, healthy advice; rather it's about fulfilling emotional neediness and coming up with avoidance strategies, etc.

For instance, your body would never say to you "I really need some ice cream." But your brain can convince you that your body will feel better or your

145

life will improve greatly if you eat some ice cream. What you really want is how the ice cream tastes (sweet), how the texture (creamy and smooth) makes you feel, and to repeat any other pleasant childhood memories (Mother's nurturing, breast feeding, etc.) you might associate with it. When we get thrown into high-stress situations, the brain takes over and in its over-stimulated state gives us some very unhealthy ideas.

Change your physiology, change your life

While the body has a lot of great ways to give you signs of what is going on, we in turn are able to control more of our health than we think. One very powerful way is by changing our physiology (e.g., heart rate, blood pressure, oxygen intake and absorption). When you begin to exercise, your heart rate increases; it has to in order for the heart to pump more blood through the body to give you the energy you need to move faster. All kinds of other bodily functions are triggered as we do things to increase heart rate and deepen the breath. As we pump the heart faster or more vigorously, we warm up the body and improve our circulation.

With many of the yoga stretches and moves you've been given, it may not seem like you are doing much, but remember that any time we lift our arms above the heart, we are doing "aerobics." The heart must pump more vigorously to move the blood up into the arms and the fingers.

Try raising the arms overhead in Mountain pose and hold them there for a few minutes. Notice how your fingers become numb and tingly and your arm muscles burn a bit. Notice your heart pumping more rapidly and your body temperature rising. Keep the breath flowing. Release the arms down slowly on an exhale.

Contrary to popular belief, doing "aerobics" doesn't mean that you have to move quickly. You can increase the heart rate simply by standing still and raising the arms over your head and holding them there for a few minutes as you breathe in and out.

As soon as you trust yourself,

you will know how to live.

-Johann Wolfgang von Goethe

AFFIRMATION: I SLOW DOWN AND LISTEN TO THE WISDOM OF MY BODY AND ITS MESSAGES.

POSE: WARRIOR TWO

- Doing this pose on a yoga sticky mat would be ideal.
- Step out to either side of your mat, feet more than a leg-length apart.
- Pivot your right heel so that your toes face to your right, while keeping your hips facing forward.
- Turn the toes of your left foot in a little bit to take the pressure off the knee.
- Keeping your hips square and facing forward, bend your right knee at a 90-degree angle or more, let it be directly stacked over the ankle or a little bit it.
- Inhale your arms up and out to the sides. Look out over the right fingertips with a gentle gaze.
- Tuck your tailbone under, feel your abs engage, and see if you can sink down with each exhale.
- Hold for 3-5 breaths. Repeat on the other side.

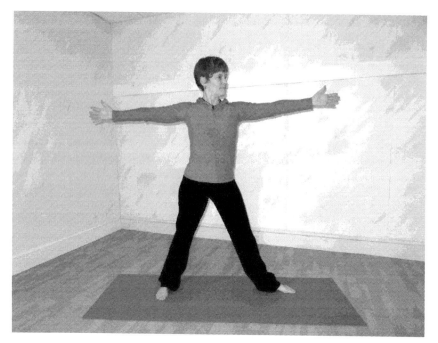

Going into Warrior 2

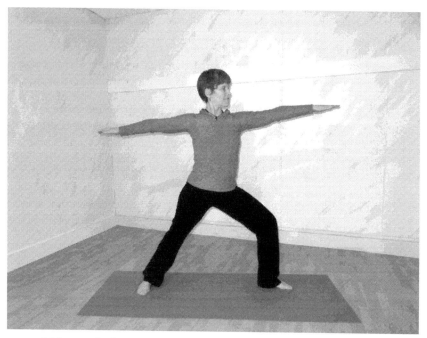

Make sure the front toes are pointed straight ahead and the knee is directly
over the ankle or a slight bit behind it.

CHAPTER 25: THE BALANCING ACT

DAY 25

Remember: Balance is not a static state. There is a flow. This is good news, because if you feel yourself off-balance then you can find your way back into balance. And even when we are perfectly balanced, there is still movement occurring inside of us through the breath and the flow of our blood and bodily fluids. We are not designed to be completely still and rigid. Learning this is a big a part of the balancing act of being alive in a body.

We all have one dominant side of our body, usually corresponding to our dominant hand. If you are right-handed, chances are your right side is much stronger than your left. That is from overuse of the right side and under-use of the left. You have built up more muscle on one side and you will be tighter and less flexible there.

By contrast, your non-dominant side will tend to be weaker and looser, but more flexible. This side may also be the one that you tend to injure more frequently. Balance is directly related to stretching and strengthening. Once you are able to feel where you are out of balance physically, you can begin to use either more stretching or more strengthening to help alleviate the imbalance.

We were born with our bodies in balance and as we grew up and took on habits, we threw off our balance, but we can always get it back. The good news is that balance is not a static state: we are constantly shifting and moving with nature as we fall into and out of balance again. Also, balancing on one side takes great abdominal strength, which is very helpful to anyone with low back issues.

Most common spinal misalignments can be traced back to muscular issues—over-developed or under-developed musculature leads to the misplacement of bony structure, in this case, the vertebrae. Muscles, tendons, and ligaments keep the bones and joints in their proper place.

AFFIRMATION: A WELL-BALANCED MIND AND BODY HELP ME TO CREATE A WELL-BALANCED LIFE.

POSE: CRANE POSE

- In standing, allow your hips to shift back and forth, rocking from side to side.
- Keep the knees loose and unlocked.
- Gradually bring more weight onto one foot and as you feel more comfortable, root one foot in standing and lift the other knee up to about hip level or as far as you are able.
- Hold here. Let your arms come up and out to the sides, like wings. Bend the wrists.
- Think "Karate Kid"—that's what this always looks like to me—without the kick.
- Breathe in and out.
- Allow yourself to wobble and wiggle as you need to and recover your balance.
- Feel the spine nice and long, shoulders relaxed, jaw loose.
- If it's a windy day and your crane falls back onto two legs, that's fine— just rock side to side again and find your perch.

- Hold for 2 to 3 breaths or longer on each side.

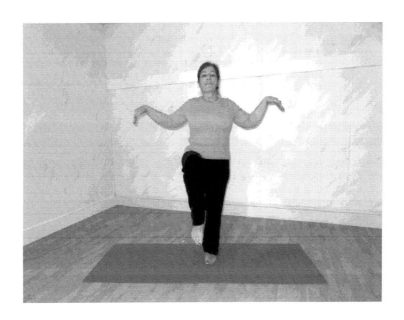

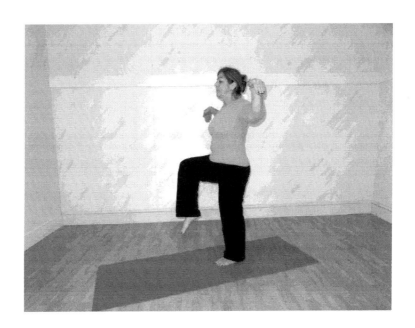

BALANCE EXPERIMENTS:

Try doing simple, everyday tasks with your non-dominant hand or side.:

1) Use your non-dominant hand to brush your teeth for one week.
2) Try eating with a fork and spoon held in your non-dominant hand for a week.
3) Cross the *other* leg over when you are sitting.
4) Use your journal pages and try to write with the non-dominant hand for one day.
5) You may think of others—kicking a soccer ball, bouncing a basketball, throwing a baseball, holding a tennis racket, pumping your gas, opening doors, use your other hand or leg.

Make notes in your journal pages: How does it feel? What is the conversation you have when you try something new? Can you feel the resistance in your body? Do you tighten up? At what point do you get used to doing the task with your non-dominant side?

Please use safety and caution around this: DO NOT apply this to the use of sharp utensils or instruments that you could hurt yourself with. The same goes for any driving habits with feet/hands—DON'T try to switch hands and feet in any way that might cause any danger to yourself or anyone else.

CHAPTER 26: LETTING GO

As discussed in Chapter 24, whenever you begin to move your body in different ways, your physiology changes. Circulation is increased as well as oxygen levels in your bloodstream. This is all **good news**. Starting with the physical body, take a moment to assess where you still need to let go -- has stiffness or discomfort shifted to new locations over these past 25 days? Use a simple breath meditation and allow whatever needs to come to the surface to do so. Make some notes in your journal about what you discover.

On a mental and emotional level, a little more detective work may be necessary. The chakra system is part of yogic and Ayurvedic philosophy, and may be very helpful in your quest to "let go."

A "chakra" (a Sanskrit word meaning "wheel") can be described as an energy center: spiraling, vibrating energy. The chakras are envisioned as these spinning energy wheels that run up and down the spine. There are 7 different chakras each associated with certain area of the body. Chakras contain life force, or in Sanskrit, *prana*, which is similar to the idea of *chi* in Chinese medicine.

If the energy of a chakra is blocked somehow, by some kind of trauma, it will not be able to spin or vibrate at the proper speed and level. This affects the localized area of the body as well as all other chakras, especially those book-ending it. When the chakras do not move, the energy is sluggish and stagnant. Breath and movement keep the prana in the chakras flowing; you just need to take a deeper breath in and out, and to move in a healing way to get the energy flowing again.

The lower back is associated with the second, or sacral, chakra. The second chakra is about relationships of all kinds -- family, friendships, romantic and sexual. It is the seat of your creative passion as well as the health and vitality of your reproductive organs. For men, this chakra relates to issues with the prostate gland or challenges with impotence and infertility; for women, this may address issues of infertility or complications with menstrual cycles, early menopause, fibroids, etc.

Exploration of the second chakra could open up interesting, possibly painful and emotionally charged issues for you to look at, specifically as they relate to your lower back pain. The lower back is responsible for supporting the whole torso; it carries a great deal of weight. If you have any sexual issues, whether physiological issues or past trauma due to rape or abuse, your lower back pain could very well be the red flag that keeps coming up and saying "please heal me, please deal with me now." If you are on this path, you are answering that call. While I am not a psychologist and cannot offer you any therapy here, I do know that movement can be a very essential part of the emotional and mental healing process.

In addition to the 7 chakras, in yogic philosophy we each have 5 koshas – energetic layers, sheaths or "bodies". The physical body is the "gross" kosha – the one that is the most solid and dense; the visible body. The next layer out from center is the prana or emotional body. The third one surrounding the first two bodies is the mental body – the seat of the intellect and the ego/personality structure. The fourth body is the wisdom body – the seat of the intuition. And finally the fifth body that is the most ethereal and the least visible, is the bliss body.

In order to truly heal your whole self, you need to recognize and acknowledge the places where you feel broken in the emotional and mental bodies as well as the physical; allow yourself to go into these places, ideally with the guidance of a teacher, to heal these other sources of trauma. Whether it's deep wounds from the past lodged in your body or limiting beliefs about yourself. Even if you're not yet sure what these old wounds are or are in the process of discovering them, opening the space for healing will help in manifesting that state.

The movement for today is one of my favorites: Breath of Joy. This combined breath and movement is great for letting go of junk—physical, mental, emotional, you name it. The description says it all and the movement delivers. Here is a chance to shed some layers.

AFFIRMATION: I REMEMBER AND FEEL THE WHOLENESS OF MY BEING AS I MOVE WITH JOY AND EASE.

MOVEMENT: BREATH OF JOY

- Stand with the feet a little wider than the hips, arms at the sides.
- On an inhale, swing the arms up overhead and stretch.
- Exhale and let the arms swing down as you come into a forward bend with a gentle squat.
- Let the arms keep going back behind you as if you are literally "throwing" or "heaving" something away. I usually tell my students to think about what you don't need any more and give it the "heave-ho."
- Allow a nice big "HA" to come out with your exhale Feel it deep down in your belly, in your gut.
- Feel the relief as you drop burdens you have been carrying around. Let go. Take out that garbage! Let go of what is not serving you…
- Inhale and swing the arms back up overhead again

- Continue this motion back and forth for 2 to 3 minutes or until you run out of steam.

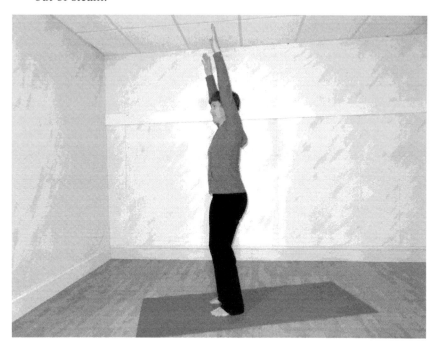

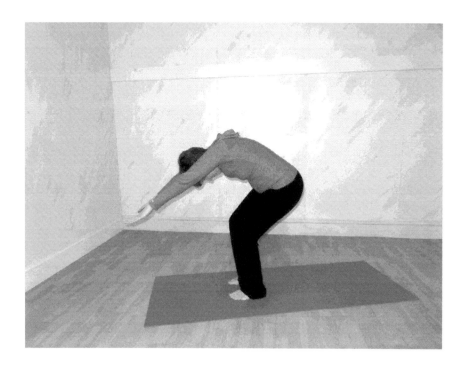

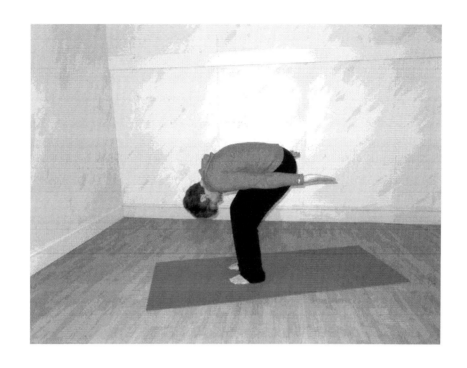

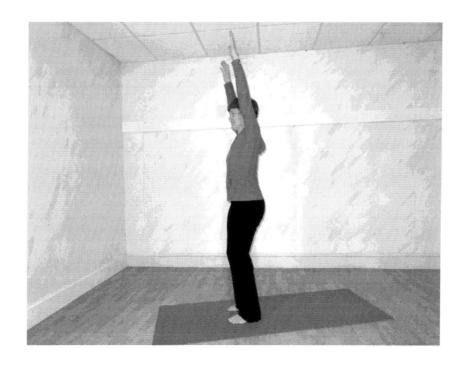

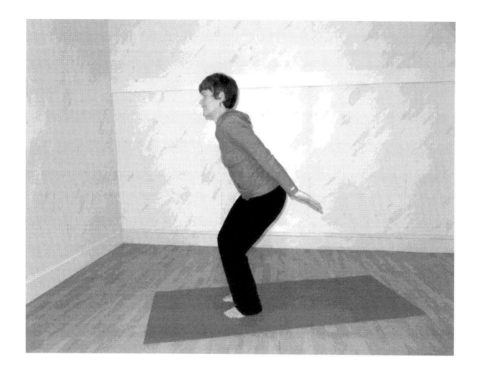

If your back is feeling tender, you can come down into a gentle squat with a straight spine and let the arms swing by your sides. This is still very beneficial, but not as intense as the forward bend.

(If you have osteopenia or osteoporosis – please do this easy version.)

CHAPTER 27: STRONG, CENTERED, FOCUSED

DAY 27

Take a few extra moments to write in your Healing Journal about these three words: **strong, centered, focused.**

What do each of these words mean to you? What image or person in your life do you think of when you hear these words—who and what embodies these qualities for you? Besides this program, are there other things you could do, other changes to your lifestyle you could make to help you cultivate more strength, center, and focus?

Our physical, emotional, and psychological bodies were meant to be in harmony and work together in synch. In other words, if I feel strong physically, I most likely feel centered and focused. If I feel very focused, then I am also aware of my strength and my center. The three are connected and each one can help to cultivate the others.

Words are powerful medicine, which is why it is also essential that even after you "end" this program, you need to keep positive words and thoughts coming in. And it's not just about the words. It's about the energetic exchange that I mentioned in Chapter 16. Open to receive the abundance prosperity; clear out the old, stagnant, negative programming and make space for healing. Take up a meditation practice and/or do some more transformational work to support your healing.

If you are breathing deeply, you are alert and therefore more aware of your surroundings—and you will be more aware of what messages are coming at you, whether from friends, family, a partner, or the television or billboards. The awareness has to come first; then you can choose to shut off some of these channels that you don't want (of course, you will need to do this gently where other human beings are involved). It's your life, your mind, and your body, so that makes it your choice.

Today is a gift. That's why they call it "the present."
--Anonymous

Remember, you always have options. You are driving this car-body of yours—take hold of the wheel and keep your focus inside and in the present moment.

AFFIRMATION: I AM STRONG, CENTERED, AND FOCUSED IN MIND AND BODY. I USE MY BREATH TO REMEMBER MY WHOLENESS – THIS IS WHO I AM.

MOVEMENT: BABY BOAT

- Start in the same position on your belly as in Half Locust.
- Use props as necessary if chests/breasts or bellies are getting in the way (use a block to rest the forehead on, etc.).

- Inhale, expanding the belly.
- Exhale, engage the abs, tuck the tailbone and feel the pubic bone push in-to the floor.
- Inhale, point the toes of both feet, and reach back, lifting both legs.
- Lift the head, shoulders, chest and arms on your next inhale.
- Exhale and release yourself back down to the floor, slowly, with control.
- Repeat this motion.

As you work with this movement and get stronger, try the full boat pose, in which your arms are held out from your sides at about 30 degrees and the head, chest, and arms also lift, after the legs are lifted. With either pose, you can hold and breathe or let the breath bring you up and down.

**Boat pose is contraindicated for Spinal Stenosis. Do Chair Dog (Chapter 19) instead and lift each leg out and up from behind you.

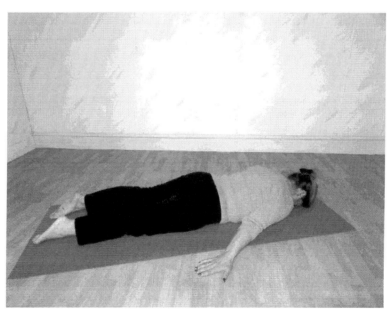

Baby boat (start)

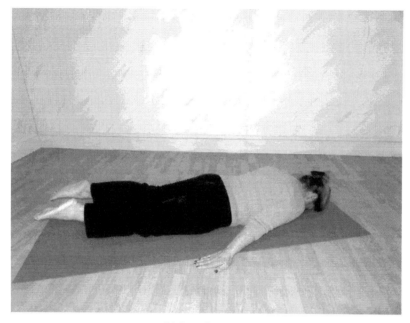

Lift legs first on an inhale,

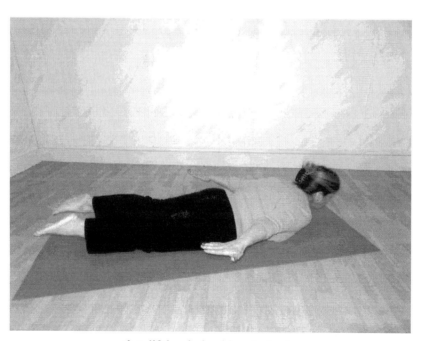

then lift head, shoulders & chest.

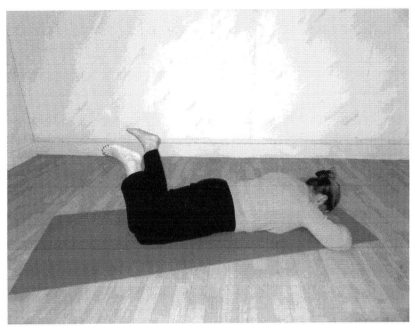

Release with windshield wipers – move feet side to side.

CHAPTER 28: ACCEPTANCE & FORGIVENESS

DAY 28

Whether you realize it or not, acceptance and forgiveness have been and continue to be a huge part of your healing process. In essence, this is where you need to start with your healing, however, sometimes it is difficult for us to hear that right off the bat and really take it in or be able to articulate it. You must have opened that space for yourself or you wouldn't have purchased this book and read this chapter, and/or completed 28 days of the program.

Whatever has happened, it can't be undone, but it's never too late to wake up, open your eyes, and take hold of the steering wheel again – make new and different, and better choices for yourself moving forward. That's what you've been doing for the past 27 days and hopefully it's become a habit for you; a habit that you now enjoy. Maybe things will keep jumping out in front of you in the road—just do your best to navigate through the obstacles and know that this enough. You are enough.

The fact of the matter is that we all must accept where we are in this moment and forgive ourselves, before we can alter our lives in a complete and holistic way. This is a very loving and compassionate thing to do. In a healthy body, mind, and spirit, it is always "the present." We may be able to use information from the past to inform our present situation or to help us in future, but the key is to stay grounded in the here and now.

When we get sick or injured, we immediately look around ourselves: "Who did I catch this from?" When we fall down, we think, "The floor was slippery—maybe I should sue." Even if you did catch your illness from someone and that floor was slippery, there is still some degree of responsibility that needs to be taken on by *you*. My spiritual teacher always reminds us that gratitude and suffering cannot exist in the same moment; just opening and shifting our energy to this loving place creates healing. It's easy to look around us at the news or even in our community and recognize that there is always someone else who is experiencing much more challenging life lessons that we are. We have so many blessings. Focus on these instead of taking the easy way out with blame.

You are just a couple of days away from "the end" of the program. I use that phrase loosely because you can go back through it as many times as you need to. If you got through 15 days and a family emergency came up, this might have thrown you off completely. It doesn't mean you have "failed" at anything. Wherever you are in this moment, let that be okay and give yourself permission to begin again. In an ideal world, I would love to see everyone stick to the 30 days the first time around and begin to see some amazing results for themselves, but sometimes, life happens and this may not be your path.

On the flip side, be honest with yourself when you see that you use the "life happens" line as a constant excuse to stay stuck in situations. We human beings can be alternately too harsh with ourselves and then do a 180 and come up with creative excuses for not taking the steps we need to in order to truly heal.

Awareness can be extremely challenging and may even seem threatening at times. You may not always like what you see about yourself when you first uncover it. You may want to blame and litigate, but ultimately, you can use all of this wisdom to free yourself from pain on many levels.

Many Westerners also prefer the quick fix of a pill to a 30-day program. We spend billions of dollars on research and development of new drugs that may be very helpful in certain situations and cases, but most of which are not designed to act as long-term solutions to a problem. And unfortunately, our society does encourage and reward the victim mentality. When you make changes to your life, it affects friends and loved ones and that can be uncomfortable for them as well as you. You may not find loads of support as you set about changing your lifestyle.

The same happens when we depend too much on the medical system and our health-care practitioners to "fix" our bodies and minds. They may have tools that can help us, but they may have long-term effects that are yet to be discovered. By taking on victim mentality, you constantly give your power away. It needs to be a collaborative effort if anything.

There is already plenty of evidence and research to suggest the urgent need for and importance of employing the complimentary therapies (CAM's), like the ones introduced here, in our everyday lives. The more we get involved in our own healing process, the more successful we will be; the more complete we will feel, and the more lasting the healing will be.

We have to get past that negative voice that seems to be everywhere we turn, not just in our own heads but also when we get together with other people who are miserable with life and themselves and like to complain (misery does love company). Maybe you have gotten yourself on a positive track, but you still hang out with the same crowd of friends, who think your 30-day healing program is "cute" or "ridiculous." You may start to notice the negative talk coming from other people: "That's rotten luck. Why don't you sue the bastards! I've heard that no one ever heals a herniated disc. Might as well let them fuse your back— nothing you can do about it." Hopefully, you are now at least aware of these voices and have gained enough strength and self-knowledge after 27 days to ignore them when they come from others and/or shut them off in your own head.

Use the many resources – therapists, teachers, books, props – offered in the Appendices here to keep your momentum going; perhaps find a support group of some sort or some positive activity or class to join. Keep re-directing yourself. The negative voice of the ego-mind is very strong, very powerful and can be very hard to break free of. You need to change the recording that's playing in your head, telling you "you can't do this" or that if you did achieve it, "it will never last." Rather, stick to the kind, compassionate thoughts, affirmations and wishes that will make your healing fluid and complete.

Write in your Healing Journal about all of the blessings in your life.

AFFIRMATION: I AM THE MASTER OF MY THOUGHTS AND ACTIONS; I CHOOSE TO CREATE HEALING IN THIS PRESENT MOMENT.

MOVEMENT: ARM SWINGS

- In standing, let your feet be a little wider than your hips.
- Gently begin to swing your arms from side to side, creating a small twisting motion in the trunk and spine.
- Let your back foot pivot on the ball to get more range of motion and protect the knee.
- Allow the hands and arms to flop against the body as you go back and forth from side to side.
- If this feels good, let yourself build up a little bit more speed and let out a "ha" sound as you go back and forth to each side.
- Imagine the spine as a wet washcloth and you are wringing out all of the toxic thoughts and feelings from your nervous system and your organs.

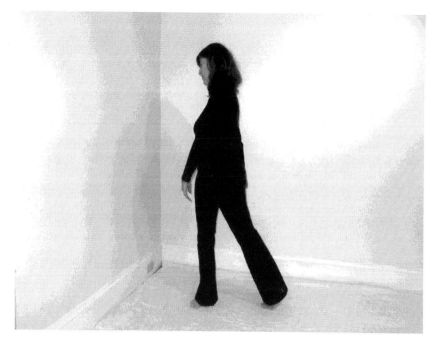

Pivot back foot

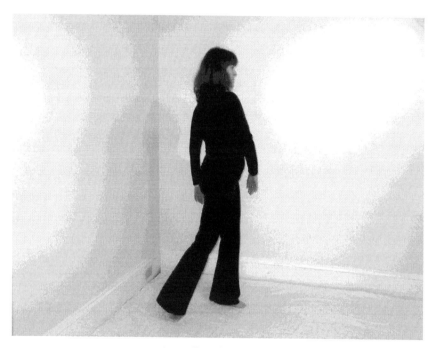

Arms flop side to side

CHAPTER 29: RE-CREATE YOUR LIFE

DAY 29

Take a moment to write in your journal pages about the opportunities you have created for a pain-free life. Do you have clearer sense of who you are and what you need to do to take better care of yourself? Write about that too. And remember the gratitude – everyday, we have so much to be grateful for.

As I have emphasized a number of times, this low back healing program is not like a conventional diet—you don't start it and then stop the routine after you achieve your goal. That is a sure way to land you right back where you started— in pain and vulnerable to re-injury. Maintaining your health is an ongoing process and it doesn't have to be that difficult. It can easily fit into your everyday routine. You've already proven that to yourself by following the program this far.

Whether you can or you can't, either way, you're right.
—Henry Ford

You have managed to change your thinking, habits, and lifestyle enough over this period of time to effect certain changes in your body and in particular your spine. The minute you abandon your routine, your spine can and will revert to its former state.

You will get stronger and feel even better as more time passes and as you continue to let this new lifestyle evolve. In order for the program to work, you must **work it** and continue to work it. All of this information will sink in deeper and become a more and more natural part of your regular routine, as simple as brushing your teeth each morning.

Give yourself credit for taking this bold step forward in your healing – choosing awareness and learning; moving and strengthening the body in gentle, effective ways that will have a lasting effect, and continuing this process.

We gain strength, and courage, and confidence

by each experience in which we really stop to look fear in the face...

we must do that which we think we cannot.

-Eleanor Roosevelt

AFFIRMATION: I BEGIN WITH GRATITUDE AND DWELL UPON WHAT I WANT TO CULTIVATE MORE OF IN MY LIFE.

POSE: GENTLE SEATED OR STANDING BACKBEND

- Sit in a straight-backed chair (no arms) and face the back of the chair (or sit on the edge and place hands on seat).
- Hold the top or side of the back of the chair for support as you gently arch and lean back (dog tilt position).
- Hold here for a breath or two and come back up. Do this 10 times.
- You can also sit facing the back of the chair with your legs coming around the sides – hold the top and gently lean back in an arch.

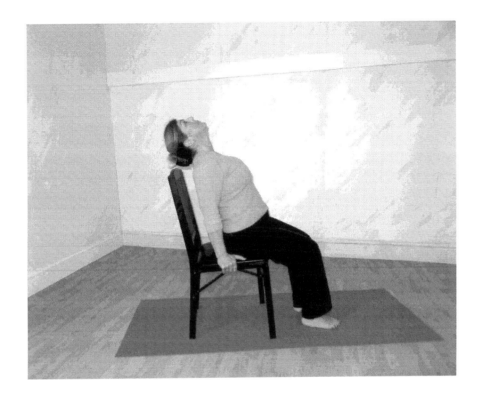

--OR –

- In a comfortable standing position, either mountain or with feet a little bit wider, find your best spinal alignment.
- You may use the foam block or sturdy cushion between your thighs if you like.
- Place your hands (palms or fists) in the small of your back for support.
- As you tuck the tailbone and engage your abs, feel the lift that begins down in your toes, runs up through your legs and the pelvic floor, navel, sternum.
- Reach up and out through the crown of the head on the inhale and on an exhale, slowly bend back, allowing the hips and pelvis to shift forward.
- Keep the knees soft and unlocked, but strong.
- If your neck bothers you, tuck it into the chin.
- Keep the knees soft.
- Hold here for a breath or two to start and let an inhale bring you back up.
- Try 5 to start or 10 if you are feeling strong.
- Feel the strength and support originating from your center.

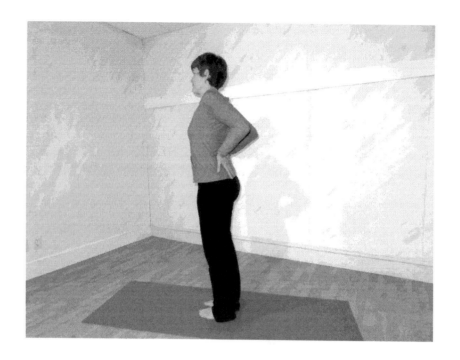

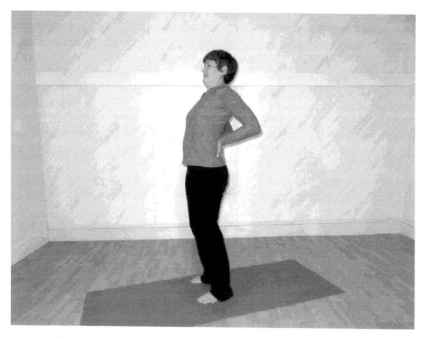

Support back, shift pelvis forward, reach with crown of head

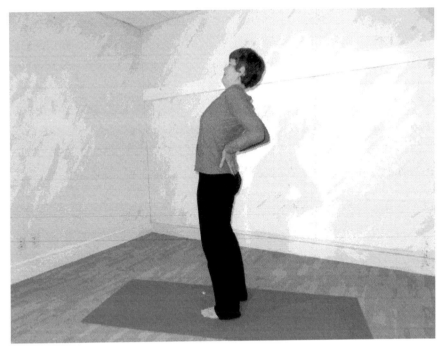

Tuck chin to support neck

CHAPTER 30: RELAX INTO WHOLENESS

DAY 30

Congratulations! This is a day of celebration. What an accomplishment! How do you feel? Please acknowledge yourself for seeing through with this commitment to your life and health. It can't hurt you to do this program as many times as you need to make the routine stick.

I have provided a blank monthly chart to print out and copy, based on the practices you have established over the last 28 days. Print it out and post it somewhere prominent where you will remember to fill it in, or carry a copy with you in your purse or business portfolio. This is your reminder. You've created a new life for yourself. This will help you to continue it beyond the 30 days.

Continue to work the program and it will become as natural as getting up each morning and taking a shower or brushing your teeth. Don't let yourself lose ground and slide back, but if life takes a turn and you do get out of your routine, notice it and quickly bring yourself back onto track again. Why make yourself work so hard and have to repeat the lessons over and over again? Stick to what you've accomplished here and enjoy your pain-free spine and new life. You may just inspire someone else to do the same.

Write in your Healing Journal about how it feels to have kept this commitment to yourself and completed the 30-day program. And it's only the beginning....now wash, rinse, repeat!

AFFIRMATION: I AM GRATEFUL FOR THIS HEALTHY, PAIN-FREE BODY.

POSE/MOVEMENT: FULL ROUTINE

- Set aside 40-60 minutes and try doing the last 29 days' worth of poses, breathing, and movements.
- End in **savasana** or with legs over a chair in **viparita karani** for as long as you can remain on your back.
- Take your time and stay connected to the breath.
- Use props as needed.
- When you complete your practice, write in your journal pages about how you feel *now,* in the present moment.
- Read over your journal from the last 30 days to assess your own journey and make note of any changes you feel.

APPENDICES:

My Healing Journal

NAME: _____

DATE: _____ DAY NUMBER: _____

_____
_____
_____
_____
_____
_____
_____
_____
_____
_____
_____
_____
_____
_____
_____
_____
_____
_____
_____
_____
_____
_____
_____

Back to Balance -- Daily Checklist

Month _____   Year_____

DAY	YOGA	BREATHING	AFFIRMATION	JOURNAL
1				
2				
3				
4				
5				
6				
7				
8				
9				
10				
11				
12				
13				
14				
15				
16				
17				
18				
19				
20				
21				
22				
23				
24				
25				
26				

27				
28				
29				
30				
31				

30 Therapeutic Movements for 30 Days

1) Modified viparita karani
2) Pelvic tilting & savasana
3) Half-frog pose
4) Child pose
5) Cat/dog (variations), plus three-part breath
6) One knee into chest, plus nadi shodhana (alternate nostril breathing)
7) Both knees into chest
8) Hamstring stretch with strap
9) Hip openers with strap
10) Half-locust
11) 10-minute routine (previous 10 movements put together), plus nadi shodhana (alternate nostril breathing)
12) Gentle supine spinal twists
13) Side rolling
14) Cobra vinyasa
15) Baby bridge/block squeeze
16) Baby sunbird
17) Gentle bounces in standing (lymphatic workout)
18) Sun breaths
19) Chair dog or downward facing dog
20) Mountain pose with block
21) Victory squats
22) Sacral massage
23) Complete rolling side to side
24) Warrior two
25) Crane pose
26) Breath of joy
27) Baby boat
28) Arm swings
29) Gentle seated or standing backbend
30) DO THE WHOLE ROUTINE: All 29 movements/poses and end in savasana or mod. viparita karani

30 Affirmations for 30 Days

1) I am fully present and grounded in this moment.
2) I gratefully take responsibility for my health and well-being.
3) I allow myself to stop and breathe – I follow my own inner rhythm as I interact with others.
4) I breathe in and expand the space inside my body, I breathe out and release more tension. I allow the breath to move me and my spine in healthy ways.
5) I ride the wave of my breath and let it guide my movements.
6) I breathe, relax, feel, watch and allow, focusing my attention inside.
7) By simply breathing and paying attention to sensation, I am becoming an expert about my own body and what it needs.
8) I make healthy, conscious choices in each moment which cultivate healing energy.
9) Knowledge is power and I enjoy learning more about my body and how it works.
10) Every day I become stronger and more flexible.
11) I trust my breath to move me and trigger the healing responses in my body.
12) I move slowly and mindfully in healthy and healing ways.
13) I open to new ways of nurturing and healing myself.
14) As I open my body and mind, I become more flexible and supple; my life flows with ease.
15) As I strengthen my core abdominal muscles, I strengthen my low back.
16) The universe is conspiring in my favor. My spine is healed and I am full of gratitude.
17) I cultivate my healing garden daily with loving, positive thoughts, deep breaths and movement from my center.
18) I breathe in positive, healing energy, I breathe out what no longer serves me.
19) I see my whole self, completely healed.
20) I honor myself and my body daily in every choice, every breath, every movement.
21) I move into a greater awareness around my everyday habits.
22) I surrender to the gift of sleep and receive its benefits.
23) My sleep is deep and sound; I welcome the rest I need to heal and wake up refreshed and renewed.
24) I slow down and listen to the wisdom of my body and its messages.
25) A well-balanced mind and body help me to create a well-balanced life.
26) I remember and feel the wholeness of as I move with joy and ease.
27) I am strong, centered, and focused in mind and body. I use my breath to remember my wholeness -- this is who I am.
28) I am the Master of my thoughts and actions; I choose to create healing in this present moment.
29) I begin with gratitude and dwell upon what I want to cultivate more of in my life.
30) I am grateful for this healthy, pain-free body.

Holistic Recovery Chart

Start Date _____**Week Number**_____

Sleeping habits

	Sun	Mon	Tues	Wed	Thurs	Fri	Sat
Time to bed							
Time awake							
Hours of actual sleep							

Eating habits

	Sun	Mon	Tues	Wed	Thurs	Fri	Sat
1st meal time							
2nd meal time							
3rd meal time							
Snack(s)							

Daily Practices for Digestion

	Sun	Mon	Tues	Wed	Thurs	Fri	Sat
Tongue cleaning							
Drink 8 oz of warm water							
Neti pot/nasal rinse							

Portions – Stay aware of these and don't overeat. Stop when you feel full, even if it means leaving food on your plate.

Beverages – Watch amount and when consumed (with meals/in between); hot or cold?

Caffeine intake -- Quit, cut-back or substitute (coffee and chocolate).

Body Type adjustments for meals --Prakriti/VPK evaluation is needed – you can do this with the help of an Ayurvedic practitioner.

Moving – Develop your daily routine for stretching & strengthening – use poses & movements chart from the book.

List of Images & Diagrams

Bibliography & Print Resources

Anatomy and Asana: Preventing Yoga Injuries by Susi Hatley Aldous

Anatomy of the Spirit by Caroline Myss

Ayurveda: The Science of Self-Healing by Dr. Vasant Lad

Balance Your Hormones, Balance Your Life by Dr. Claudia Welch

Creating Health by Deepak Chopra

How Did I Get Here? By Dr. Barbara DeAngelis

I Have Become Alive by Swami Muktananda

It's All in Your Head: Change Your Mind, Change Your Health, by Mark Pettus, M.D.

The Key Muscles of Hatha Yoga by Ray Long, M.D.

Live Pain-Free Without Drugs or Surgery by Lee Albert, NMT

The Omnivore's Dilemma by Michael Pollan

Pay Attention for Goodness Sake by Sylvia Boorstein

Relax and Renew by Judith Lasater, Ph.D., P.T.

The Relaxation Response by Herbert Benson, M.D.

Self-Awakening Yoga by Don Stapleton, www.nosarayoga.com

The Wisdom of Yoga by Stephen Cope

Yoga for Wellness by Gary Kraftsow

The Yoga Sutras of Patanjali translated by Chip Hartranft

Yoga and the Quest for the True Self by Stephen Cope

Yoga and Ayurveda by Dr. David Frawley

Yoga Teachers' Toolbox by Joseph and Lilian Le Page

You Can Heal Your Life by Louise Hay

"Decreased Melatonin Production Linked to Light Exposure", Blask DE, Brainard GC, Dauchy RT, Hanifin JP, Davidson LK, Krause JA, et al. 2005. Cancer Res 65(23):11174-11184.

Online Resources

American Chiropractic Association, http://www.amerchiro.org

American Psychological Association,

       http://www.apa.org/monitor/may05/physician.html

American Viniyoga Institute, www.viniyoga.com

The Chiropractic Journal, Orthotic support

       http://www.worldchiropracticalliance.org/tcj/2003/mar

Habits of the Heart: The Lungs

       http://www.smm.org/heart/lungs/top.html (excellent graphics and videos)

Holistic Online

       http://www.holisticonline.com/Remedies/Sleep/sleep_ins_relaxation.htm

Kripalu Center, www.kripalu.org

The Laser Spine Institute, www.laserspineinstitute.com

Medline Plus Medical Dictionary,

       http://www.nlm.nih.gov/medlineplus/mplusdictionary.html

Metro Health, www.metrohealth.org

National Osteoporosis Foundation, www.nof.org

Network Spinal Analysis, http://www.wiseworldseminars.com

Podiatry Today, Orthotics, http://www.podiatrytoday.com/article/1400

Positional release therapy, http://www.cihh.net/overservicesprt.htm

Spine Universe, http://www.spineuniverse.com/

U.S. Department of Labor, Occupational Safety & Health Administration,

       http://www.osha.gov/SLTC/etools/computerworkstations/

WebMD.com, http://dictionary.webmd.com/

Practitioners & Instructors

Lee Albert, NMT (positional release therapy), http://www.leealbert.com

Vidya Carolyn Dell'uomo, http://www.opentolife.net/

Stephen Cope, http://www.kripalu.org/presenter/V0000065

Dr. Barbara De Angelis, www.barbaradeangelis.com

Devarshi Steven Hartman, http://www.stevenhartman.com

Julie Gudmestad, http://www.gudmestadyoga.com/index.htm

Brahmani Liebman, http://www.rivertownyoga.com

Sudha Carolyn Lundeen, http://www.sudhalundeen.com

Sara Meeks, www.sarameekspt.com

Hasita Agathe Nadai, http://www.yogagaia.com/ & www.rivertownyoga.com

Dr. Paul Muller-Ortega, www.bluethroatyoga.com

Don & Amba Stapleton www.nosarayoga.com

Products & Props

Relax-o-back (sturdy wedge cushions) http://www.relaxobak.com

Sara Meeks programs and products, www.sarameekspt.com

Master Caster Lumbar Support Cushion (adjustable) – search for this online;
    many stores carry it

*Many other types and styles of lumbar support cushions are available online, but make sure the foam is good quality, durable and sturdy. There are also many different wedge cushions available, though the foam may not be as dense and sturdy as the Relax-o-Back.

YOGA SUPPLIES -- Search Hugger Mugger or Gaiam online, or check your local Target, Walmart, TJ Maxx, Marshall's or other discount store for a better deal on these items: foam yoga blocks (3 inch), strap, yoga mat, bolster, Mexican or sturdy wool blanket, eye pillow.

10 Easy Ways to De-Stress Everyday

In our culture, we experience stress in any number of different ways. Stressors are the things which trigger our stress or panic response and then these responses may manifest in our lives through our bodies, minds and/or our feelings and reactions. Below is a list of small, but significant things you can use to keep stress at bay!!

1) **SLOW DOWN and BREATHE DEEPLY.** Take a moment to stop and notice what is going on inside of you. Slow, deep breathing quiets the mind and calms the nervous system, slows the heart rate, oxygenates the blood and relaxes muscle tension.

2) **FOCUS ON JOY!!** Slowing down will help make you more sensitive to the joyful things going on all around you, especially children laughing; birds singing; the sounds of the natural world outside; any kind of music.

3) **TAKE TIME TO GIVE THANKS**. Before you go to bed each night or when awaken in the morning, make a gratitude list of what you are grateful for in your life. Name 5 or 10 people and things.

4) **GO ON A MEDIA DIET**. We always worry about body weight & what we feed ourselves through the mouth, but the eyes and ears are also receiving and digesting. Watch what you allow in and how much of it. Turn off TV, computers - spend time with friends and loved ones. When you use your cell phone, call someone you haven't spoken to in years and surprise them!! Use media devices for positive effect.

5) **GET OUTSIDE IN NATURE**. Weather-permitting, do your best to get outside for some fresh air. Walk slowly, watch and listen to what the natural world is doing around you.

6) **SPEND TIME WITH YOUR FRIENDS AND FAMILY.** Make an effort to schedule time for the people in your life who are important to you. The greatest gift you can give anyone is your time and attention.

7) **MAKE QUIET TIME FOR YOURSELF.** Likewise, it is just as important to let yourself have time for reflection, meditation or prayer. Take 5 or 10 minutes in the morning and evening to sit quietly and breathe.

8) **SPEND TIME IN SERVICE TO A CHARITY OR AN INDIVIDUAL IN NEED**. Be clear about your intention here – do it because you know it's the right thing to do. Don't expect to gain anything from it… enjoy how good it feels to give your time to those in need. "Extend love. Experience Joy."

9) **FOCUS ON THE GOOD NEWS!!!** We can't control the events of the world, but we can control which ones we focus on. Search for what is good in the world and send out our good wishes and blessings to all who are suffering, instead of focusing on the suffering and fear.

10) **BE GENTLE WITH YOURSELF** and others. We must learn how to create peace within ourselves and our own lives before we can be truly peaceful with others and create peace in the world.

<u>10-Minute Desk Routine</u>

Take at least one minute for each move/pose or less if you only have 5 minutes.

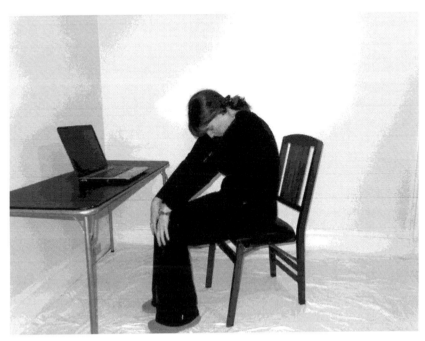

Seated cat stretch

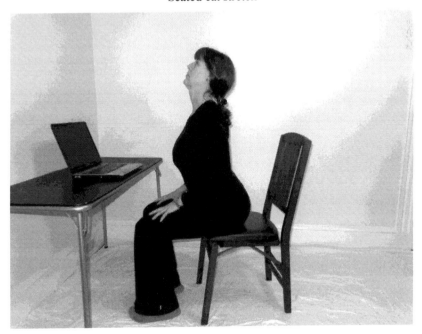

Seated dog tilt

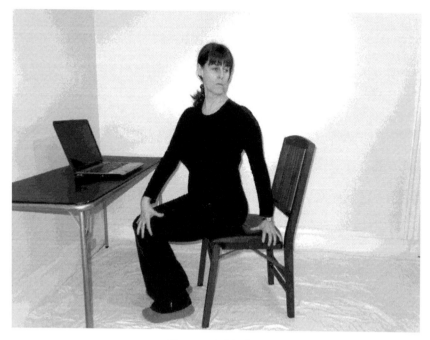

Easy seated twist

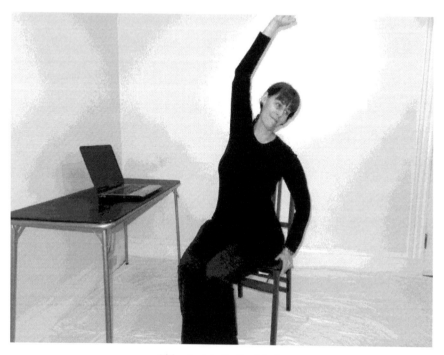

Side stretch (both sides)

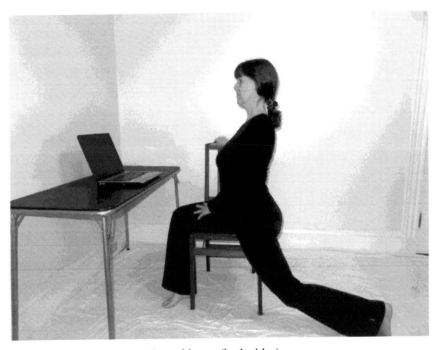

Seated lunge (both sides) –
sit on edge and turn first before extending back leg

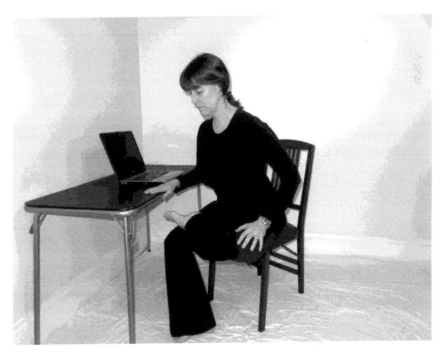

Chair half lotus -- bend forward from hips,
do both sides (watch knees!)

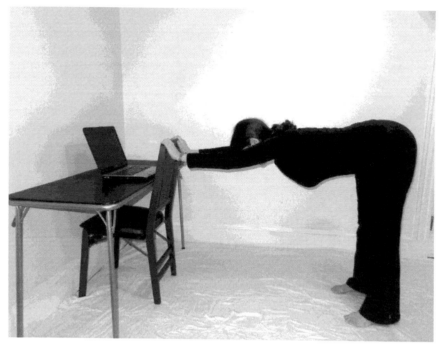

"Chair Dog" -- flat back, keep head in line with spine and hips

Holistic Pain Management – Daily Checklist

<u>When you wake up, before getting out of bed…</u>

Take 10 long, deep breaths; spend a few moments in silence, breathing and noticing sensation in your body; notice how your lower back feels.

Connect to your emotions and feeling state – release unwanted thoughts and feelings – anything negative; inhale deeply and on the exhale LET GO of anything that does not serve you.

Lie back down for a moment and give your knees a hug, roll head and neck side to side.

Sitting on the edge of your bed, do some cat/dog stretches (Chapter 12, page 60) and foot stretches (flex and point the feet), shift the hips from side to side.

Take another moment to think about what you are grateful for in your life.

<u>Throughout your day….</u>

Once every hour or so, take time to pause in your "busy-ness" and take a few long, deep breaths to reconnect with sensation in your body.

Remind yourself not to stay locked in any one position too long; stand up from time to time and shake out arms, legs, hands/wrists. If the neck is tight, roll it gently from side to side; shift weight from one leg to the other, do some little stretches (they need not be "yoga"!). Whatever feels good.

Take lots of "gratitude breaks;" focus on what is good and positive in your life.

<u>Before going to sleep…</u>

If you tend to get leg cramps at night or have plantar fascitis, stretch out those calves before you get into bed.

In bed, hugs your knees into your chest and do some gentling rolling side to side. Make sure you let your body stretch and move as it needs to before lying down and while you are getting comfortable in a lying down position.

Once again, take time to give thanks for your day, your life, your health and anything else in whatever way is appropriate for you.

Ergonomic Guidelines for Sitting and Standing:

At your computer....

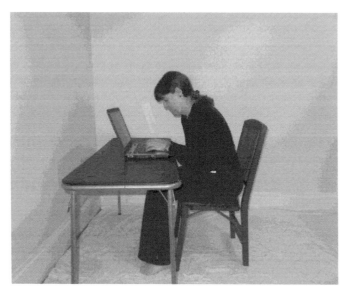

Rounded posture shown, or sometimes leaning back with arms extended too far.

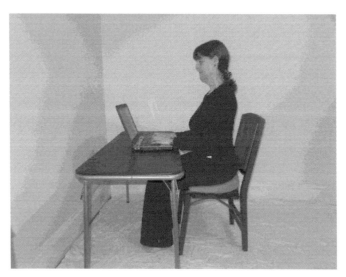

Ergonomically correct posture – ear, shoulder, hip all line up;
elbows at right angles, feet on floor; using a wedge cushion
(on a desktop, screen could be propped up higher for the neck)

Sitting....

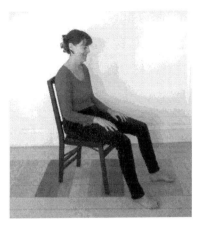

Typical posture, rounded back

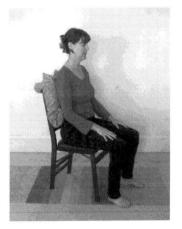

Use a rolled up pillow for support

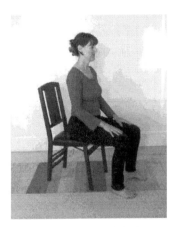

Or sit on edge of chair,
feet flat on floor

Standing…

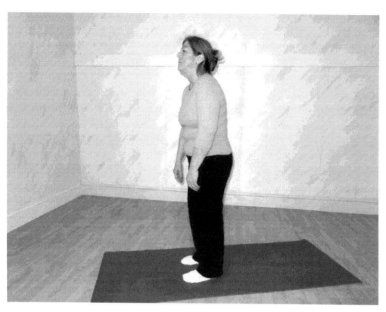

Typical posture – spine taking on the weight of the head

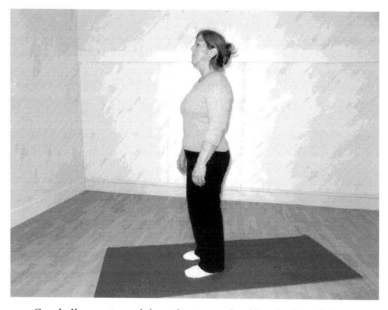

Good alignment – pelvis under torso, shoulders back and down

Energy Centers of the Body (Chakras)

CHAKRA	LOCATION	SANSKRIT NAME	COLOR	FOCUS
FIRST -- ROOT	BASE OF SPINE/ PELVIC FLOOR	MULDHARA	RED	ALL IS ONE; TRIBAL POWER, BELONGING, SAFETY
SECOND – SACRAL	JUST BELOW THE BELLY BUTTON	SVADISTHANA	ORANGE	RELATIONSHIPS; SEXUALITY; HONOR ONE ANOTHER
THIRD – SO-LAR PLEXUS	BETWEEN BELLY BUT-TON & HEART	MANIPURA	YELLOW	PERSONAL POWER, WILL, HONOR ONE-SELF
FOURTH – HEART	MID-CHEST BY THE HEART	ANAHATA	GREEN	FORGIVENESS, COM-PASSION, HEALING, UNITY
FIFTH – THROAT	THROAT	VISHUDDHA	BLUE	CREATIVE EXPRES-SION; COMMUNICA-TION
SIXTH – THIRD EYE	BETWEEN THE EYEBROWS	ANJA	INDIGO	INTUITION; VISION; IMAGINATION
SEVENTH – CROWN	TOP OF THE HEAD	SAHASRARA	VIOLET OR WHITE	FAITH; WITNESS CONSIOUSNESS; EN-LIGHTENMENT

Understanding Hormones

When we think of hormones, we usually think of estrogen and testosterone, but there are many other hormones, not related to our reproductive systems, which play some very important roles in our everyday wellness.

Cortisol is produced in the adrenal glands and is responsible for the following tasks:

- Regulation of blood pressure
- Proper glucose metabolism
- Insulin release for blood sugar maintenance
- Immune function
- Inflammatory response

Normally, cortisol levels rise during the early morning hours and are highest about 7 a.m. They drop very low in the evening and during the early phase of sleep. However, if you sleep during the day and are up at night, this pattern may be reversed. If you do not have this daily change (diurnal rhythm) in cortisol levels, you may have overactive adrenal glands. This condition is called **Cushing's syndrome.**

Although stress isn't the only reason that cortisol is secreted into the bloodstream, it has been termed "the stress hormone" because it's also secreted in higher levels during the body's **'fight or flight'** response to stress, and is responsible for several stress-related changes in the body.

Slight increased levels of cortisol have some positive effects:

- A quick burst of energy for survival purposes
- Enhanced memory
- A burst of increased immunity
- Lower sensitivity to pain

While cortisol is an important and helpful part of the body's response to stress, it's important that the relaxation response be activated so that functions can return to normal following a stressful event. Unfortunately, in our high-stress culture, complicated by our generally poor posture, the body's stress response is activated so often that it doesn't always have a chance to return to normal, resulting in a state of chronic stress. You may have heard the expression "tired and wired" – that best describes this state.

Adrenaline is another hormone produced in the adrenal glands. The adrenals are located directly above the kidneys in the human body, and are roughly three inches in length. The kidneys are located near the lower thoracic and upper lumbar region of the spine. Low back pain can be a sign of kidney disease.

Adrenaline stimulates the heart-rate, dilates blood vessels and air passages, and has a number of more minor effects. Just as with cortisol, adrenaline is naturally produced and released into the body in response to high-stress or physically exhilarating situations. This is an early evolutionary adaptation which allows us humans to better cope with dangerous and unexpected situations. With dilated blood vessels and air passages, the body is able to pass more blood to the muscles and get oxygen into the lungs more quickly, increasing one's stamina for short bursts of time.

Norepinephrine (or noradrenaline) is another hormone released from the adrenal glands when they are active. In a healthily functioning human, approximately 80% of the released substance is adrenaline, and the other 20% is norepinephrine. Norepinephrine is also a **neurotransmitter.**

It can be useful to 'work off' the adrenaline that has been released into your system after a particularly stressful situation. Our ancestors handled this naturally through fighting or other physical exertion, but in the modern world, high-stress situations often arise that that involve little physical activity. If high amounts of adrenaline accumulate in the body with no way of being processed, this can result in insomnia, agitation and restlessness. A regular regimen of physical exercise (cardio) which raises the heart rate can help to process the excess adrenaline.

Insulin is another hormone, and like many hormones, it's a protein. Insulin is secreted by groups of cells within the pancreas. The pancreas sits behind the stomach and has many functions in addition to insulin production.

The pancreas also produces digestive enzymes and other hormones.

Carbohydrates (sugars) are absorbed from the intestines into the bloodstream after a meal. In response to an increase in blood sugar, insulin is secreted by the pancreas. Most cells of the body have insulin receptors which bind the insulin as it circulates. When a cell has insulin attached to its surface, the cell activates other receptors designed to absorb glucose (sugar) from the blood stream into the inside of the cell.

Without insulin to help us breakdown sugars, we could eat lots of food, but literally end up "starving". Many cells cannot access the calories contained in the glucose properly without the help of insulin. This is why Type 1 diabetics who do not make insulin can become very ill without insulin shots.

More commonly these days, people develop **insulin resistance** (Type 2 Diabetes) rather than a true deficiency of insulin. In this case, the levels of insulin in the blood are similar or even a little higher than in normal, non-diabetic individuals. However, many cells of Type 2 diabetics respond sluggishly to the insulin they make and their cells cannot absorb and process the sugar molecules very well. This leads to blood sugar levels which run higher than normal. Occasionally Type 2 diabetics will need insulin shots but most of the time other medication and lifestyle and diet management will work well.

Melatonin is a naturally occurring hormone found in most animals, including humans, and some other living organisms, including algae. Melatonin is important in the regulation of the circadian rhythms of several biological functions. It is also a powerful antioxidant with a particular role in the protection of nuclear and mitochondrial DNA. In humans, it is I produced in the pineal gland.

Bright light inhibits melatonin production by inhibiting neural activity in the pineal gland. Darkness has the opposite effect stimulates the production of melatonin by increasing neural activity to the gland. The light-translating abilities of the pineal gland may explain why it is known as the "Third Eye." The third eye chakra sits between the eyebrows, with the pineal gland located in the brain just behind this external area.

The use of melatonin as a drug can synchronize our circadian rhythms to environmental cycles and can have beneficial effects for treatment of certain insomnias. Melatonin is normally released at night (in the dark) as we sleep.

The incidence of breast cancer is five times higher in women living in industrialized nations compared to those living in developing countries, and female night shift workers have particularly high rates of the disease. [1]

---

[1] Decreased Melatonin Production Linked to Light Exposure, Blask DE, Brainard GC, Dauchy RT, Hanifin JP, Davidson LK, Krause JA, et al. 2005. Cancer Res 65(23):11174-11184.

Understanding Neurotransmitters

Endorphins are among the brain chemicals known as **neurotransmitters**, which transmit electrical signals within the nervous system. Endorphins can be found in the pituitary gland, in other parts of the brain, or distributed throughout the nervous system. They are produced in the pituitary gland (the "master gland" of the endocrine system) which is located at the base of the brain and is about the size of a pea.

Stress and pain are the two most common factors which lead to the release of endorphins. When endorphin levels are increased, we feel less pain and fewer negative effects of stress. They act similarly to drugs such as morphine and codeine, however, the activation of the opiate receptors in the brain does not lead to addiction or dependence.

Endorphins are thought to be modulators of the "runner's high" or "the zone" that athletes experience with prolonged exertion and movement. Endorphins also help to control appetite, release sex hormones, and boost our immune response.

Stimulating foods like chocolate or chili peppers, can also cause an increase in the secretion of endorphins. The release of endorphins explains the comforting feelings that many associate with chocolate and the craving for it when we are under stress. Studies of acupuncture and massage therapy have shown that both of these techniques can stimulate endorphin secretion. Sex is also a major trigger for endorphin release. And on the other end of the spectrum, the practice of meditation can increase the amount of endorphins released in your body.

Serotonin is another important neurotransmitter in the functioning of the cardiovascular, kidney, immune and digestive systems. Low serotonin levels are usually seen in people with depression.

<u>Glossary</u>

Ayurveda -- the sister science to yoga; a form of self-healing and life-style management that has been practiced for more than 5,000 years in India. Ayurveda instructs us in how to live in harmony with nature and within our own bodies. It addresses everything from physical, mental, emotional and spiritual issues to our eating and sleeping habits. Its basic premise is that all health and disease begin in the digestive tract and that we must maintain a proper amount of digestive fire (agni) in order for optimal health.

Bulging disc – a disc which extends outside the space it should normally occupy. The bulge may make the disc look a little like a hamburger that's too big for its bun. The part of the disk that's bulging is typically the tough outer layer of cartilage. Usually bulging is considered part of the normal aging process of the disk and is common to see on MRIs of people in almost every age group.

Central Nervous System (CNS) – the brain and the spinal cord only. See Peripheral Nervous System (PNS).

Chakra – Sanskrit word used in yoga and Ayurveda, meaning "wheel." Used to describe the "energy centers" of the body which are aligned with the spine from root (tailbone/pelvic floor area) up to the crown of the head. Typically, there are 7 chakras, but some yogic philosophies believe there to be 12. Each wheel is vibrating or spinning at a certain velocity. Ideally, all chakras should be open and vibrating at their highest frequency for optimum mind-body-spirit health.

Degenerative Disc Disease (DDD) -- is not really a disease but a term used to describe the normal changes in your spinal discs as you age. The discs act as shock absorbers for the spine, allowing it to flex, bend, and twist.

The loss of fluid in the disc means losing height and you have less of a shock absorber in place. The body responds to the loss of padding by creating bone spurs which can cause a great deal of compression on the nerves.

While disc degeneration is a normal part of aging and for most people is

203

not a problem, for certain individuals a degenerated disc can cause severe chronic pain if left untreated.

This degeneration process can be accelerated by injury and herniations which do not heal properly or at all. The most common areas for degeneration are the lumbar and cervical regions of the spine.

Erector spinae -- These muscles run the length of the spine on each side and help the abdominal muscles support the entire torso and maintain good posture. The erector spinae muscles are not single large muscles but rather groups of smaller muscles and tendons. The erectors stretch from the tailbone to the top of the rib cage with the individual muscles attaching at various points along the way.

Dosha – A term used in Ayurveda to describe the elemental qualities (vata, pitta and kapha) in our human constitution; these are distributed in different ways and amounts within each person and there are usually one or two dominant qualities within each of us, though it is possible to be "tri-doshic" and have all three in equal amounts. Vata describes the elements of air and space; pitta, describes the elements of fire and water and kapha, represents the elements of earth and water in the body.

Gluteus medius – A smaller muscle that attaches the top of the iliac crest of the pelvis to the top of the femur (greater trochanter). This muscle steadies the pelvis so it does not sag when the opposite side is not supported with the leg.

Herniated disc – This results when a rupture in the tough outer layer of cartilage allows some of the softer inner cartilage to protrude out of the disk. The protrusion of inner cartilage in a herniated disk usually happens in one distinct area of the disk and not along a large component of the disk, which is more typical of a bulging disk. Herniated disks are also called slipped or prolapsed discs. Bulging discs are more common. Herniated discs are more likely to cause pain, but many people have bulging discs or herniated discs that cause no pain whatsoever.

This condition most frequently occurs in the lumbar region and results in loss of disc height and fluid, and more pressure on the nerves, etc. A herniation will usually heal naturally with therapy and lifestyle changes.

Hormone -- A chemical substance produced in the body that controls and regulates the activity of certain cells or organs. Many hormones are secreted by special glands, such as thyroid hormone produced by the thyroid gland. Hormones are essential for every activity of life, including the processes of digestion, metabolism, growth, reproduction, and mood control. Many hormones, such as neurotransmitters, are active in more than one physical process.

Kosha – Sanskrit word used in yoga and Ayurveda, referring to the 5 layers, sheaths, coverings or bodies of our Self from the densest, physical body (Annamaya kosha) to the most subtle, bliss body (Anandamaya kosha). Ideally, we want to balance and heal all of our koshas – physical, emotional, mental, wisdom/intuitive and bliss.

Kyphosis – An exaggerated outward curvature of the thoracic region of the spinal column resulting in a rounded upper back, usually a result of hunching over and caving in the chest over a period of time.

Lordosis – An exaggerated forward curvature of the lumbar and cervical regions of the spinal column, i.e. "swayback," where the tailbone is tipped up and back to an extreme and the pelvis is tipped forward causing a more pronounced curve in the lower back. This requires the upper body to over-compensate by positioning the torso too far forward, in front of the hips. When the vertebrae are not stacked in their natural "S" curve, this throws off the whole alignment of the spine and can cause all kinds of problems.

Osteoarthritis – A condition in which the cartilage that protects and cushions the joints breaks down over time. Eventually, the bones-formerly separated by the cartilage-rub against each other, resulting in damage to the tissue and underlying bone and causing painful joint symptoms. Osteoarthritis is the most common form of arthritis and is a major cause of disability in older adults. It most often affects the spine, fingers, thumbs, hips, knees, or toes.

Osteoporosis -- A condition that especially affects older women and is characterized by decrease in bone mass with decreased density and enlargement of bone spaces (porous); bones become brittle and more likely to break due to loss of bone mineral density (BMD). The disease is most common in the spine, hip and wrist.

Osteopenia – A condition in which the bone mineral density is lower than normal, but not low enough to be classified as osteoporosis. It is a good wake-up call to get before you are diagnosed with full-blown osteoporosis.

Parasympathetic Nervous System -- The part of the involuntary nervous system that serves to slow the heart rate, increase intestinal and glandular activity, and relax the sphincter muscles.

Peripheral Nervous System (PNS) – All of the nerves outside of the brain and spinal cord, which connect the central nervous system (CNS) to sensory organs, such as the eye and ear, and to other organs of the body, muscles, blood vessels, and glands. The peripheral nerves include the 12 cranial nerves, the spinal nerves and roots, and the autonomic nerves. The autonomic nerves are concerned with automatic functions of the body, specifically with the regulation of the heart muscle, the tiny muscles that line the walls of blood vessels, and glands.

Piriformis - A muscle that lies deep within the gluteal region and is covered by the gluteus maximus. It originates at the front surface of the sacrum and passes through the greater sciatic notch to attach to the top of the thighbone (femur). The piriformis crosses the sciatic nerve and can be a cause of sciatica.

Quadratus Lumborum – A large, dense muscle that connects the bottom of the ribcage (12th rib) to the top of the pelvis (iliac crest) and also attaches to Lumbar vertebrae 1 through 4. This muscle is difficult to stretch and release and a very tight QL can frequently be misdiagnosed as a lumbar spine issue.

Sciatic Nerve - The sciatic nerve is comprised of five nerves. It is formed on the right and left hand side of the lower spine by the combination of the fourth and fifth lumbar nerves and the first three nerves in the sacral spine.

Each nerve exits the spine between two vertebral segments and is named for the segment above it. The five nerves group together on the front surface of the piriformis muscle (in the rear) and become one large nerve – and the longest one in the human body. This nerve then travels down the back of each leg, branching out to provide motor and sensory functions to specific regions of the leg and foot.

Sciatica – A compression of the sciatic nerve, causing localized pain in the gluteal area and/or shooting pains down the legs.

Scoliosis -- A lateral curvature of the spine; another common misalignment which can be treated effectively with a program of stretching and strengthening of the erector spinae muscles which hold the spine in place. This can either develop out of bad habits of leaning to one side over time or there can be scoliosis present at birth. In babies, the spine is still soft cartilage and the bony structure of the spine will not be fully formed until beyond the 16th year of life, so it's best to catch and treat this early on.

There has been a great deal written about how baby walkers and playpens can hinder the proper spinal and neurological development of children. Babies need to creep and crawl – they need to learn how to pull and push themselves up and around, strengthening the spine naturally. If this does not occur, the vertebrae may not develop correctly or may fuse together in the lower spine.

Scoliosis or lordosis is more likely to occur in children who were not allowed to crawl as babies. And back braces prescribed for children to treat scoliosis usually end up weakening the spinal muscles further and causing even more discomfort and a greater problem. Make sure you get 2nd and 3rd opinions before putting your child in a brace or taking other drastic action.

Spinal Fusion – A surgical fusion of two or more vertebrae for remedial immobilization of the spine. Typically a bone graft is taken from the hip to replace the lost disc height and shift the vertebrae back into place. Bones spurs will eventually develop over the bone graft, causing arthritis. .[2]

---

[2] www.laserspineinstitute.com

Some of the possible fusion complications include:

- Allergic reaction to the implant materials
- Bending, breakage, loosening, and/or migration of the implants
- Bleeding, which may require a blood transfusion
- Bone fracture or failure to fuse
- Bone formation that is abnormal, excessive, or in an unintended location
- Bowel, bladder, or gastrointestinal problems
- Damage to nearby tissues
- Death
- Fetal development complications
- Infection
- Pain or discomfort
- Paralysis or other neurological problems
- Postoperative changes in spinal curvature, loss of correction, or disc height
- Respiratory (breathing) problems
- Scar formation or other problems with the surgical incision
- Sexual dysfunction
- Side effects from anesthesia or the surgical approach
- Spinal cord or nerve damage
- Tears of the dura (a layer of tissue covering the spinal cord)
- Vascular problems other than bleeding

Spinal stenosis -- The narrowing of the space where the spinal cord is housed (the spinal canal). Essentially, the spinal cord and nerve roots are squeezed or compressed. This used to be called "creeping paralysis" because it comes on slowly and results in numbness and deadness in the extremities (legs if it's lumbar, arms if it's cervical), eventually resulting in total loss of motor or muscular use. Most people complain of weakness or have problems falling because the numbness strikes them suddenly as they walk or stand. (Most full extensions are contraindicated for stenosis; modifications may help.)

Spondylosis – Osteoarthritis and any of various degenerative diseases of the spine.

Spondylolisthesis – The forward displacement of a lumbar vertebra on the one below it and especially of the fifth lumbar vertebra on the sacrum producing pain by compression of nerve roots

Subluxation -- From the Latin word "luxare" meaning "to dislocate," is the same idea as spondylolisthesis – the vertebrae have slipped out of alignment

– the only difference being that spondylolisthesis usually occurs in the lumbar spine, whereas subluxations or misalignments may occur throughout the spine.

Sympathetic Nervous System -- A part of the nervous system that serves to accelerate the heart rate, constrict blood vessels, and raise blood pressure. The sympathetic nervous system and the <u>parasympathetic nervous system</u> constitute the <u>autonomic nervous system</u>.

Trapezius – The large muscle which connects the neck (beginning at the base of the skull) to the shoulder girdle and wraps around to the collarbone in front. There are 3 parts to it – the upper, middle and lower regions. The upper trapezius is the muscle on top of your shoulders that becomes very sore. The trapezius helps us to move the head forward and back and the neck side to side; it also allows us to rotate the shoulder blades and move them up and down. They also help us with breathing, and they do look a lot like flattened "wings" on our back when you see an anatomical drawing.

About the Author

Raven Sadhaka Seltzer, M.A., E-RYT-500, is a yoga therapist and wellness consultant, trained and certified through The Kripalu Center for Yoga and Health and the Yoga Alliance. She is also a Reiki Master, trained in the Usui Method. Although her specialty is low back and neck pain relief and recovery, Raven has worked successfully with clients suffering from everything from plantar fascitis and fibromyalgia, to those with thyroid conditions and hip and knee surgery rehabilitation. She has also worked with cancer survivors through their treatment and remission.

Raven has practiced and studied the medical science of Ayurveda for a number years and trained at the Kripalu School of Ayurveda. She also has an extensive background in expressive movement/dance, music and creative writing. She holds an M.A. in writing and filmmaking from the University of Southern California and a B.A. from Mount Holyoke College in Russian Studies.

Her yoga path began in 1981 with basic hatha yoga classes. Along the way, she also trained in Chi Kung, Tai Chi and Kung Fu and became a licensed massage therapist in Los Angeles in 1995.

Raven has been teaching yoga and offering this spinal healing program to private clients and classes since 2003. She is an alternative healthcare provider through several major insurance companies and offers a discount for subscribers for private sessions and consultations.

For a private consultation (in person or by phone/Skype), ergonomic evaluation, or to book one of Raven's "Back to Balance" workshops at your studio, school or place of business, please contact info@selfhealingsolutions.com. Raven's website is www.selfhealingsolutions.com .

About the Models

Stephanie Laverdiere is an Occupational Therapist, specializing in early intervention. She has been working at Children's Hospital of Boston for the past 10 years and has been studying yoga with Raven since 2010. Yoga therapy has helped her rehabilitate a frozen shoulder condition.

Marian Murphy has been a teacher in the Boston Public School System for the past 21 years. She has been studying yoga with Raven for 4 years. Yoga has helped her to de-stress, relax and increase her energy level. It was also helpful in rehabilitation from ankle surgery.

Made in the USA
Lexington, KY
22 September 2013